The Cappuccino Principle~

Health, Culture, and Social Justice
in the Workplace

The Cappuccino Principle~

Health, Culture, and Social Justice in the Workplace

Merle Jacobs

de Sitter Publications

LIBRARY AND ARCHIVES CANADA CATALOGUING IN PUBLICATION

MERLE JACOBS

THE CAPPUCCINO PRINCIPLE: HEALTH, CULTURE AND SOCIAL JUSTICE IN THE WORKPLACE / MERLE JACOBS

INCLUDES INDEX.

ISBN 1-897160-26-7

Cover design by Aloma Lively. Lively Designs

All remuneration from this book to the author shall be donated to the
Toronto Youth for Humanity.

de Sitter Publications
http://www.desitterpublications.com

The ability to understand and recognize how things have an affect on us and others allows for a choice of how we resolve to live our lives.

/

~ DEDICATION ~

James Alexander Jacobs

Francisco Antonio DeLaMaza

The design for this cover was based upon material and key points made in the book, *The Cappuccino Principle*. The images were chosen specifically to reflect the disparity in hiring practices prevalent in our society in various areas of the workforce. The images of racialized minorities encased in white shows that we are one world and need the support of the dominant group. It is also used to show that cooperation and understanding is needed from the dominant group to be able to rise to the top. The smaller images provide the viewer with the idea of the helplessness of those portrayed. Some of the minority groups have the ability to rise; however, they still don't make it to the top of the cream of positions. Those positions are traditionally given to the dominant group. Even within the dominant group, gender plays a role that determines where one sits in the cream of the cappuccino cup.   ~ Aloma Lively, Artist

Table of Contents

Foreword

"Nursing, like a cappuccino – white on top, brown on the bottom –requires stirring up."

Stirring the Cappuccino: Toward Racial integration in Nursing

The above quotation bedecked the recent report to the Canadian Race Relations Foundation (CRRF) submitted by the Centre for Equity in Health and Society (CEHS) (Hagey et al. 2005). A cup of cappuccino being stirred serves up the opening image of the CEHS website (www.BeforEQuality. com) a play on words that announces "Be For Equality!" and "Make sure you have EQ or Emotional Quotient before working on Quality!"

This foreword touches upon six of the recommendations in the Participatory Action Research (PAR) report published by the CRRF entitled *Implementing accountability for equity and ending racial backlash in nursing.* The report argues that if the dismantling of institutionalized racism in research, education and practice is to occur, some form of accountability for racial discrimination, exclusion and segregation should be present in various domains: interpersonal encounters with co-workers and services with clients, as well as administrative policy and procedure including those of unions and professions and state mechanisms such as provincial and territorial human rights commissions and the Charter of Rights and Freedoms, and much needed employment equity legislation.

Using nursing as a retrospective case example, Jacobs in *The Cappuccino Principle* re-reads a survey, email tracking, and participatory observation notes from 142 staff nurses who were not divided into racialised and non-racialised informants. She uncovers a multitude of critiques by nurses who are acutely aware of power relations including those of race relations, a topic Jacobs had not actually itemized in her questionnaire circulated in a purposive sample in the hospitals the participants worked at across the GTA.

The findings in *Cappuccino Principle* dramatically resonate with those from the CEHS study that involved 200 racialised nurses and their supporters who exploited participatory action research to challenge policy and practices. The key finding by CEHS is the perception that practices are characterized by avoidance of accountability for equity and oblivion to the apparent cultural rule uncovered during the research: in a racist society one does not necessarily have to hold oneself accountable to racialised people or agendas for racial equality. Moreover, CEHS found massive disagreement or conflict about what to do about this state of affairs.

In both studies and others done on the topic, racialised nurses reported being targeted and set-up to take extra work during nurse shortages and job transfers or job termination during job shortages following restructuring in Ontario healthcare, but were at a loss about what to do about this pattern. The pattern suggests the cappuccino principle serves a labour strategy of having compliant, silent, racialised nurses to hire whom you can lay off if you don't need them.

Recent years have seen a shift away from interest in race relations in favour of addressing the patterns of systemic or endemic racial disparities. As early as 1985 adverse or systemic effects of racism have been acknowledged in Canada, for example in a Supreme Court decision (OHRC v. Simpson-Sears 1985 (2 S.C.R. 536); see Black 2004). Beck, Reitz and Weiner (2002) have, however, lamented that the 1996 amendments to the Canadian Human Rights Act and federal Equal Employment Act have actually weakened accountability for systemic discrimination. In the same year Ontario's Equal Opportunity Plan rescinded the first provincial employment equity act in Canada, putting the onus on individuals, employers, unions, professional and other tribunals to address discrimination, with the result that enormous sums of health care dollars are being used to settle racial disputes out of view of the public eye with few accountability mechanisms in place to either prevent or de-escalate conflict (Hagey et al. 2005).

Although racial domination and disparities are manifestations of systemic racism, nurses both in Jacobs' and in the CEHS study tend to experience the problem of racism as a relational one, viewing accountability as a dimension of relationship. The generalized fear of backlash for broaching issues of racism acts as a deterrent to questioning and problem solving to restore substantive equality. Jacobs' analyses emphasize the dilemma that nurses experience in whether to speak up and face predictable negative consequences or to face equally predictable negative consequences by suffering in silence. She offers the strategy of organizing and advocating and her final chapter is a very practical primer on how to advocate.

Jacobs asks early on, "how do we construct the culture of collegiality?" She illuminates how conflict and collegiality play hand in hand in the responses to the economic and political pressures that organize nursing work regulated by hand maidens who are the wives, mothers, daughters and friends of the white males who regulate the health care system and society. Hence, the cappuccino image helps to illustrate nursing's resistance to changing the whiteness at the top and the otherness in the lower echelons of nursing. Whiteness and otherness are cultural categories that mediate structured relations and determine privileges and disadvantages, (Hagey and MacKay 2000).

The recommendations in the CEHS report have helped to set the direction of CEHS as a research and advocacy organization that envisions expanding into anti-racism education and policy initiatives. The Ontario Human Rights Commission (OHRC), the Health Council of Canada (HCC), the Ontario Nurses Association, the Registered Nurses Association of Ontario, the Canadian Nurses Association, Ontario Ministries of Education, and of Colleges, Training and Universities, and of Health and Long Term Care, the Nursing Secretariat, the Joint Commission on Hospital Accreditation, the Canadian Association of Schools of Nursing, the provincial and territorial councils on nursing education programs, research funding bodies, hospital associations, regulatory and professional bodies, in-service orientation programs, faculty development programs and so on are subjects for lobbying initiatives. Many of these are discussed at length in the *Cappuccino Principle*.

Ongoing participatory action research and advocacy within CEHS by Aboriginal, migratory and other racialised nurses use strategies of lobbying, negotiation, supporting each other, demonstrating, requiring hearings to redress grievances and complaints concerning various of these offices.

The CEHS recommendations pertain to legislation as well as to political and administrative policy and education. They have implications for funding, research, change in political processes and reporting routes, continuous quality improvement technologies, curriculum, accreditation, dissemination of demographic data, development of best practices, registration mechanisms, composition of regulatory panels, and development of ethnoracial competencies. (See the glossary.)

Jacobs' model advises moving past the inter-personal domain of behaviour and the domain of organizational cultures to intervene in structures of the state and the administrative apparati that it oversees. Despite a healthy critique of technologies of work surveillance in her earlier work (see Visano 2006), Jacobs has assisted the CEHS network in asking that equitability and accessibility be employed as elements of quality, i.e., as criteria for measures that can monitor and promote equity and support diversities in nursing work and health care with diverse populations.

The following is a brief elaboration upon the recommendations put forth by the partisan branches of the CEHS network to address the cappuccino principle in systemic disparities. That is, total consensus was not required to put forth a recommendation.

Recommendations by the CEHS seeking accountability for systemic disparities

1) The Health Council of Canada that emerged following the Romanow Commission was seen as a body that could introduce accountability mechanisms to monitor the costs associated with systemic racial disparities in health and health care and set guidelines for equity practices. The Romanow Report Recommendation 3.2 states that *"On an initial basis, the Health Council of Canada should establish benchmarks, collect information and report publicly on efforts to improve quality, access and outcomes in the health care system"* (Romanow 2002, p. 248).

It is recommend that the Health Council of Canada:

- Monitor the racial disparities in health and health care and require interventions to correct them
- Require process and outcomes reports on equity programs for health care workers and consumers
- Monitor the number of health care dollars spent on defending discriminatory practices and set mechanisms to ensure freedom from racial discrimination, harassment, set-up and backlash in organizations responsible for health.
- Promote equal access and participation in organizations responsible for health including the provision of interpreter services and removal of barriers for racialised people and invisible minorities.

2) The Ontario Human Rights Commission under section 29(g) of the Code can investigate situations when problems continue without numerical data collection and such data are required to be obtained by the commission who are competent to interpret such data. Nursing is seen as resisting research on racism. Nursing leaders (defined as top level managers) were seen as

lacking in diversity and not interested in understanding racialist phenomena or gaining competencies. Very few (N=2) attended any of the think tanks or other venues publicized for knowledge transfer during the PAR. Moreover, in a survey sponsored by the College of Nurses of Ontario, nurses were asked "would you like to participate in research in the future" and since a large proportion answered "no", research on nurses with the support of the College is now conveniently prohibited (CEHS diaries, July, 5, 2005).

It is recommended that the Ontario Human Rights Commission:

- Initiate an investigation into the systematic discrimination against racialised nurses as well as all designated groups protected under the code with respect to education and employment in the health care system. The investigation should take account of discrimination, harassment, and procedures for redressing grievances and complaints.

3) The Centre for Equity in Health and Society became incorporated during the PAR research; it is a coalition of nursing associations and community agencies with a vision for achieving equal access and participation in organizations responsible for health. Its mission is to promote policies and programs for accountability towards equal access and participation through research, advocacy, recognition, and leadership development. Participants felt that current leadership training for nurses is devoid of knowledge about anti-racism and therefore diversity in leadership is impeded as evidenced by the Statistics Canada 1991 Census showing that white nurses in Ontario have twice the chance of moving into management positions as their racialised counterparts (Nestel 2000). Participants also reported the lack of formal anti-racism curriculum in schools resulted in explicit racism from colleagues and supervisors during the SARS crisis. Participants belonging to unions reported the widespread problem of member-to-member racial disputes pertaining to discrimination, systemic racism and lack of ethnoracial competencies among nurses (Meeks 2003).

It is recommended that the Centre for Equity in Health and Society:

- Convene dialogues in nursing on the overt racism from patients, colleagues and supervisors experienced by nurses of Asian and Filipino descent during the outbreak of SARS and how to prevent

racist behaviours in future.
- Collaborate with unions that negotiate nurses' contracts to sponsor conferences that discuss innovations addressing member-to-member racial disputes.
- In partnership with university research units, evaluate curricula and develop and disseminate new knowledge on ethnoracial competencies and achieving diversity in leadership.
- Establish a leadership academy that holds training workshops for negotiating the implementation of anti-racism policy and practice in support of ethnoracial competencies.

4) The College of Nurses of Ontario was seen as lacking in diversity in its review panels and administration of programs making for poor representation of the diverse communities of clients and of nurses. (The mandate of the College is to protect Ontario patients receiving nursing care through the regulation of standards of practice.) The racialised and migratory nurses felt they were more vulnerable than others for being reported to the College and racialised managers felt they were more likely to be harassed by their superiors and those in their charge than other nurses are. As participants learned about cases where nurses had to defend themselves under charges by the College, they observed that the proceedings did not lend themselves well to accounting for the nature of racism or understanding the vulnerabilities of racialised nurses and patients. Although transformative justice is a relatively new accountability process, it is used successfully by the Urban Alliance on Race Relations (CEHS diaries, March 12, 2004). By convening discussions that bring out perceptions and concerns not admitted when strict legal rules of evidence are followed, for example, prohibiting the use of the word "racism", more meaningful, fair and learning-based proceedings may be possible (see Hagey et al. in Jacobs 2006).

It is recommended that the College of Nurses of Ontario:

- Introduce transformative justice proceedings to handle allegations where a racial dispute is evident between a client and a nurse.

5) The Canadian Association of Schools of Nursing accreditation arm is responsible for reviewing nursing school curricula and requiring changes to conform to standards. The criteria that schools must follow in preparing for review are undergoing change so now is an opportune time to introduce

antiracism principles and guidelines. Moreover, the Aboriginal Nurses Association of Canada with other bodies has recently completed a report recommending the inclusion of Aboriginal students, staff and faculty in nursing education and content pertaining to Aboriginal health in the curriculum (Author 2002).

It is recommended that the Canadian Association of Schools of Nursing:

- Require evidence of recruitment and strategies for retention of Aboriginal, racialised and non-visible minority faculty and students.
- Require evidence of anti-racism being practiced in the lived curriculum.
- Require evidence of ethnoracial competencies among faculty, staff and students.

6) Research funding bodies could play an important role in partnership with professional and regulatory bodies in facilitating comparative data on racialised and non-racialised nurses and clients and their experiences in the health care system. Moreover, they could encourage research and development of equity assurance tools as part of quality assurance performance review and assess the impact on perceptions of fairness and other indicators such as absenteeism, mental health and retention of staff and mortality and morbidity of patients. Statistics Canada in particular could make available data comparing occupational groups according to Aboriginal status, ethnicity, first language, visible minority identity and so on. As pointed out by the OHRC in its recent report, *Policy and Guidelines on Racism and Racial Discrimination: "It is a common misperception that the Code prohibits the collection and analysis of data identifying people based on race and other Code grounds. Many individuals, organizations and institutions mistakenly believe that collecting this data is automatically antithetical to human rights"* (Author 2005, p.44.). The OHRC study has a number of recommendations touching on this issue of collecting and analyzing data in order to monitor equality and promote equity. See also Author (2003). The CEHS urges all employers to study the 2005 OHRC document and appreciate how their organizations can be strengthened from the principles of fairness that both their clients and their employees will benefit from if they implement its guidelines.

The results of stirring?

At this writing, young professionals, many of them nurses are celebrating the apology given to families of those immigrants from China who paid an unfair Head Tax, not required for immigrants of European extraction. It was reported that women in the Chinese Canadian community have spent years of organizing to finally obtain the apology and some compensation (CEHS diaries: Wu 2006). The organizing that nurses, mostly women are undertaking to bring about accountability in the form of apologies and compensation for unfair treatment should not be underestimated.

At this writing, the central executive of the Ontario Nurses Association, the largest union that negotiates contracts for nurses, (45,000 strong) is in dispute with one of its locals (097) and the dispute is deemed to be racial by members of the local executive which have been under trusteeship by the central in order to manage conflict (Donkoh 2006). The *Cappuccino Principle* should be taken seriously, since overt racial conflicts can only become more frequent and more explosive in a society that denies the issues and ignores finding solutions to problems.

Nursing is a profession deemed as fundamental to society and is at a crossroads. Nurses can take the lead in promoting knowledge on racial conflict, pathways to equity and diversity in leadership and develop a working model for dismantling the ethnoracially-based segregation in our microcosm of society (Ornstein 2000). Conversely, we can continue with patterns of racial domination, marginalization, exclusion, 'problematization', containment, and other modes of unacknowledged conflict that are the hallmarks of the cappuccino principle that impedes the potential for collegiality among nurses who are asking for racial integration based on equality not on unequal assimilation. Other occupations and professions too, can learn from this polemical case study. Nursing can become attractive to new recruits when principles of social justice replace the cappuccino principle.

Foreword by Dr. Rebecca Hagey
Professor of Nursing
University of Toronto

References

Author. 2002. *Against the odds: Aboriginal nursing. National Task Force on Recruitment and Retention Strategies*. Ottawa: Health Canada.

Author. 2003. *Guidelines on collecting data on enumerated grounds under the Code*. Toronto: Queen's Printer: Ontario Human Rights Commission. www.ohrc.on.ca.

Author. 2005. *Policy and Guidelines on Racism and Racial Discrimination*. Toronto: Ontario Human rights Commission. www.ohrc.on.ca.

Black, B. 2004. "The human rights process and race discrimination complaints." Special issue on racial discrimination, racism and human rights. Canadian Diversity/ Diversite Canadienne. A publication of the *Association for Canadian Studies*. Vol. 3(3): 22-24. http://www.ohrc.on.ca.

Beck, J. H., Reitz, J. G., and Weiner, N. 2002. "Addressing Systemic Racial Discrimination in Employment: The Health Canada Case and Implications of Legislative Change." *Canadian Public Policy*. Vol. 28(3): 373-394. (March).

CEHS Diaries. 2004. Confidential archived diary entry, March 12, 2004. Diversity Health Practitioner's Network meeting.

CEHS Diaries. 2005. Confidential archived diary entry, July 5, 2005.

CEHS Diaries 2006. Historical archive June 26, 2006 re: Personal communication with Betty Wu, Public Health Nurse regarding the "apology committee" headed by Susan Eng and Amy Go who are asking for compensation to families whose members paid the head tax.

Donkah, S. 2006. "Nurses speak out." *Canada Extra*. May 25-31; Vol. 4(21): P1, p5.

Hagey, R. and MacKay, R. 2000. Qualitative research to identify racialist discourse towards equity in nursing curricula. *International Journal of Nursing Studies*. Vol. 37: 45-56.

Hagey, R., Jacobs, M., Turrittin, J., Lee, R., Purdy, M., Chandler, M., Cooper Brathwaite, A. and Das Gupta, T. 2005. "Implementing accountability for equity and ending racial backlash in nursing." Toronto: Canadian Race Relations Foundation. www.crr.ca.

Hagey, R., Lum, L., Turrittin, J., and MacKay, R. 2006. "How the profession of nursing can achieve ethnoracial safety through transformative justice." In M. Jacobs and S. Bosanac, Eds. *The Professionalization of work*. Whitby: de Sitter Publications pp. 144-164.

Meeks, D. 2003. *Deconstructing Romanow*. Concurrent session at the Canadian Race Relations Foundation Award of Excellence Symposium, entitled Racism: Breaking through the denial. March 28. Sheraton Hotel, Toronto, Ontario.

Nestel, S. 2000. "Proletarianization and Racilization: Constructing the Nursing Labour Force in Ontario." Toronto: Sociology and Equity Studies in Education, OISE/University of Toronto (unpublished).

Ornstein, M. 2000. "Ethnoracial inequality in Toronto: Analysis of the 1996 Census." Prepared for the Chief Administrator's Office of the City of Toronto.

Romanow, R. 2002. *Royal commission on the future of health care in Canada*: Final report. Ottawa: Health Canada.

Visano, L. 2006. Foreword: "Cultures of coercive credentialism." In M. Jacobs and S. Bosanac, Eds. *The Professionalization of work*. Whitby: de Sitter Publications, pp. xvii-xviii.

Websites
www.crr.ca
www.BeforeQuality.com

Glossary

Ethnoracial competencies: Skills manifested by healthy discourse practices (*e.g., advocacy, bridging, consensus building, negotiation to remove barriers, holding individuals and organizations accountable) that* integrate anti-racism principles and strategies in decisions and relationships. Can also refer to broad based people skills that transact equity pertaining to age, class, disability, gender, race, sexual diversity and so on (Meeks, 2003)

Preface

It is rare to find a book that skillfully weaves together empirical data, sociological analysis and broad knowledge about the nursing profession in such a pleasantly readable package, a format that delivers original and multiple insights about contemporary occupational nursing cultures. The contents of *The Cappuccino Principle* reflect a wonderfully broad panorama of the field of nursing studies. It challenges with remarkable insights and analytic skill what has become the increasingly prevalent liberal and multicultural rhetoric regarding race, gender and equality in the workplace. The scope, objectives and the sheer amount of new evidence it brings together, its command of very disparate literatures and debates make it an impressive piece of work, and clearly worth reading.

This book is a welcome and provocative set of themes that extend our thinking about institutional roles, rules, and collegiality, theoretically and programmatically. As a result of her sustained interdisciplinary work, Dr. Jacobs evaluates the impact of the occupational culture of the nursing profession on the internal distribution of resources as mediated by race. Most mainstream studies on the nursing profession – usually the only available texts – tend to adopt a simplistic framework of "problems and prospects", whereas this pioneering scholarship assembles compelling data regarding the unhealthy contradictions perpetrated by the professional/collegial values and routine practices. Here, however, we discover an innovatively thorough and enlightening study of the social reproductions of institutionalized injustice, notably the ethos of white superiority. The silent voices of the "racialised" others speak loudly to the dominant culture of compliance that is protected in self-serving professions. Rather than simply debunk mythologies, Dr. Jacobs appeals to academics and practitioners alike to consider seriously those themes that have been woefully overlooked in studies of professions—social justice. Justice, an increasingly significant theme in public policy and program, provides a direction that is long overdue in addressing micro conflicts within macro contexts.

Admittedly, this clearly courageous study, interested in making the work world more humane, will be too easily dismissed as rancorously iconoclastic. The book is surely a thought provoking contribution to social science scholarship in terms of its eye-opening and well-grounded discussions of controversy. The ideas set forth will generate discussion, from practitioners to social justice advocates. There is much food for thought in these pages, shedding light on the relationship between the disadvantage of democratic accountability and the arrogance of professional independence. The book is a thoughtful examination of the reasons why social justice proposals are so easily discarded in a profession ostensibly oriented to principles of care.

Nursing, like so many other professions, can profit greatly from the impressive intellectual framework and policy elaborations of this study. In all, this book is a welcome, and very much needed addition to the sociologies of profession/work/ occupations, health studies, and social justice. Reform is warranted. Human rights organizations and academics would be well advised to draw important insights from this and other similar studies, in the hope of developing generalized principles of social reform. Anyone interested in the nursing profession especially, and health policies culture generally, should read this book. Indeed, given the implications of applications of exclusion, this work deserves a wide reading. Dr. Jacobs' rewarding analysis of equal protection for disadvantaged groups will stimulate further thought and research, and could be read profitably in conjunction with other intersecting forms of exclusion. As Martin Luther King Jr. admonished, "...our lives begin to end the day we become silent about things that matter."

Preface by Dr. L.A. Visano,
Professor, York University

Acknowledgements

This project is indebted to the many staff nurses who provided me with their narratives and experiences- the voices from the margin, thank you so very much. To name each of you would take pages, so I express to each of you "without the staff nurse we would not have a vibrant nursing profession." My colleagues in psychiatry, you demonstrated collegiality in actions and words. The many hours we spent discussing social inequality provided me with several insights towards understanding the structural components which often left out the interest of the disadvantaged. You are also my friends and gave of your time amid many cups of tea to discuss issues raised in this book, I want to say thank you for your support and for ideas relating to race and ethnicity. Each one of you makes a difference in my life.

To the racialized managers and racialized staff nurses thank you for sharing your experiences with me. You trusted me enough to share uncomfortable feelings and interactions. I would not have understood the true meaning of racism and the different forms it takes when discussing social justice in the context of women's work. I must take this opportunity to acknowledge my nursing classmates from the *Branson Hospital School of Nursing*. You provided me with my first understanding of collegiality. To you, my sisters, I will always be grateful for the friendship and warmth provided me as a student nurse and a new Canadian. This enduring friendship is not only collegial but where each one of us contributes to the well being of the whole group.

A note of gratitude to Ray Morris, Livy Visano and Tania Das Gupta. I first met Professor Ray Morris in an undergraduate statistical course. Ray has always been a wonderful example as a mentor and supervisor. You opened my mind to race, class and gender and how oppression effect's our everyday life. I am grateful for the many insights as well as your support over the years. To Professor L. A. Visano thank you for your friendship and collegiality, and for encouraging me to "just keep writing." Your work in the area of justice inspired several insights in the area of social and economic justice. I thank you for sharing insightful comments as well as your critical imagination which help guide my research. Thank you for writing the Preface. The work of Professor Tania Das Gupta in 'Racism and paid work' helped me situate and build understandings in the area of racism in nursing. Her categories were useful to me in understanding several behaviours and identifying them as racism within the healthcare system. I know the discussions I had with you helped me appreciate many of the issues debated in this book.

For the review of the manuscript and their excellent suggestions I thank the following scholars: Robynne Neugebauer, Linda Muzzin, Hira Singh, and Jane Turrittin. They provided helpful advice and pedagogical directions. I remain indebted to them for their time, the critical insights gained and their continued assistance.

I give special thanks to Professor Rebecca Hagey, a scholar who practices social justice, for agreeing to write the Foreword. Her suggestions were incorporated and I thank her for taking the time to direct me to a number of useful sources. I could not have completed this book without the encouragement and the indispensable advice and assistance of Althea Prince, a scholar and friend who read every word and provided extremely important suggestions.

My friend, Aloma Lively, always believed that I would succeed in doing this project and helped this undertaking in tangible ways. I wish to acknowledge her magnificent art illustration and cover design as well to say thank you for the skilful copy-editing.

Dr. Robert Higgins provided me with his expertise in understanding my survey results, thank you for your help and support. I want to thank Stephen Dobson for his editorial assistances and for incorporating the suggested changes. Malo Pandit for your excellence assistance, I want to thank you for the insight into how human resources are used and misused within the health sector.

To the wonderful staff at work: Paula Yanofsky, Mavis Griffin, Joni Kingsley, Loretta Fiorini, Lucy Oliveira and Rosanna Moretti, your constant support and kindness to faculty, students and staff makes our department a special place to work. I will always remember your kindness. To the students in my classes who contribute to my learning experience in the area of social justice I owe a tremendous debt. Your continued support and communication with me contributes to my teaching experience. Thank you for your valuable feedback.

I owe particular thanks to Shivu Ishwaran and de Sitter Publications. I am truly grateful for your quick and enthusiastic reaction to my manuscript. I wish to acknowledge the mission and history of de Sitter Publications which is committed to progressive projects. Your steadfast belief in my work encouraged the completion of this book. For the title, I have to acknowledge the scholarly writing 'Implementing Accountability for Equity" which first employed 'The Cappuccino Principle' in a Canadian Race Relations Foundation project.

To the peoples of Burma whose suffering and struggles since the 1960s are not on the front pages, I will not forget you or your fight for justice and democracy. I want to thank the organizers and participants of the July 15th 2006 Conference on Burma in Toronto for including my remarks on social justice and making me welcome. I will always be indebted and appreciate my roots in Burma.

My father, (the late) James Jacobs, provided me with values relating to human rights and demonstrated concern in social and economic justice. My parents taught me to respect everyone and provide for those in need. I want to pay special tribute to my mother, Doreen, for helping me complete my goals. Growing up in Burma, my three brothers and extended family provided encouragement as well making a safe community in spite of government oppression. All these experiences have inspired and helped me in my academic pursuits. Now dispersed throughout the world I am grateful for their ongoing support.

Finally, I would like to thank Francisco who provided support when I was a student nurse encouraging me to complete the program and never give up. His insightful comments and belief in this project is greatly appreciated. As well, his observations and suggestions have contributed to this book in so many ways. His fight for justice and equity helped when I lacked certainty. He was hugely encouraging, provided confidence and advocacy when problems arose which helped me produce new understandings in the area of social justice. Thank you for always supporting my work.

Introduction

This book has two objectives. First, the research evaluates the environment that contributes to the culture of the nursing profession within which inter-actions occur and how these issues relate to collegiality, conflict, and social justice. The research also examines the use of resources within the work environment, and discusses how the redistribution of these resources relates to social and economic advantages, and disadvantages. Flowing from that discussion is an examination of how power structures involved in the distri-bution of occupational advantages impact on the way the system operates. This will illuminate some of the obstacles that racialised nurses face within the health care system (see Berhadl and Moore 2006). It will be made clear that the intersections of race and gender allow for double jeopardy to occur with regard to social and economic justice in the work environment. Thus, racialised women can be and are targeted because they are women, and also because of their minority status.

Secondly, I will examine collegiality at the staff nurse level, and discuss how this group—the largest group in a female dominated profes-sion—behaves, and what action can be taken at the grassroots level. I rely on documented information on the nursing profession within the Ontario health care system, as well as the data collected specifically for this study. Canada is proud of its ethno-cultural diversity, and claims that it is one of the best countries in the world in which to live. Social and economic discrimination exists in Canada, however, and it is not a new topic for scholarly discourse. In his memoirs, Bromley Armstrong (2000) provides a picture of struggle against all types of racism and the public policies designed to alleviate the problem. In documenting his experience as a rail-way porter, and his life in general, Armstrong describes how political and civil society has changed since his arrival in Canada in 1947. His discus-sion focuses on overt and covert forms of racism in Canadian society, as well as on the importance of the federal government's enactment of the Canadian Multiculturalism Act in 1985.

Since organizations have developed policies on sexual harassment and racism to reduce and outlaw racist behaviours in the work environment, there has been some improvement. In spite of this, however, we notice that occupational structures, unions, and government systems are still very white at the top (see Porter 1965; Ornstein 2000). It is clear that the dominant group feels a sense of ownership of top-level positions, and racialised and ethnic minority candidates see this acted out in a number of ways. They find themselves excluded from short-lists; their achievements are discounted, and their qualifications need to be superior to those of their white counterparts in order for them to carry weight.

Unspoken in this type of occupational racism is what is viewed as "essential knowledge" and professional activities that are usually Eurocentric. These standards are based on the yardstick of a few power brokers who create job postings, and who place their mentored white protégées into available jobs.

Work is a part of most of our lives, and success in this area makes a difference in how we succeed in society at large. The title of this book is suggestive of my intention: that being, to lead to greater understanding of social and economic justice within occupational structures. Specifically, the focus of the book is women's work within the profession of nursing. The terms "professionalism" and "collegiality" are both positive aspects of many occupations, and are current concerns within the nursing profession. Yet, often, managers use them as strategies to discredit 'the other'. I believe that using collegiality to highlight the contradictions within this occupational structure will provide a framework and an overview of structural, systemic racism, as well as other abuses that frontline workers experience.

My interest in collegiality arose out of discussions on professionalism among nursing leaders that occurred during the nineteen-nineties. When interviewing staff nurses, I learned, however, that racialised nurses were experiencing harassment, rather than collegiality from the administration, and from other nurses. Some racialised nurses who experienced racism within the professional structures and work environment filed a number of complaints at the Ontario Human Rights Commission (Papp 1994; Collins et al. 1999). These cases helped to establish that we can no longer state that the experience of racism is not systemic within nursing, and is occurring as isolated incidents.

Another study (Modibo 2004) demonstrated that hospital administrators made distinctions between Black, Brown, and White nurses. Modibo concludes that such categories appeared to be linked to another distinction: that is, country of origin, and ethnicity. He suggests that white managers and co-workers draw on ideological constructs (racialised, gendered, matriarchal, and patriarchal relations of the society) to support the systemic workplace segregation of Black nurses in Toronto's health-care institutions (112).

Apart from racism, my research demonstrates that staff nurses experienced verbal and physical abuse, sexism, bullying, as well as 'feeling' that management was passing down to them the cutbacks that were occurring within the hospital. They were angry, and complained about the hospital environment, the lack of respect for their roles from their peers, the physicians, and especially from nursing management. A major concern was the change in staff nurse/patient ratio, while management swelled its own ranks with new positions. At the same time, management blamed the government for lack of funding, while staff nurses viewed this as the pervasiveness of inequality within the work environment, and within the profession of nursing in general.

Staff nurses within the health care system are the largest group of frontline workers, yet they do not always fully exercise their power when injustice occurs. The contradictions inherent in their profession reflect the process described in policies, mission statements, and objectives, versus outcomes and practices.

When examining social justice, I discuss social and economic rights within occupational structures, as well as within a profession. Social justice is seen then, as not being about individual rights but focuses on fairness and equity for classes of people. Social, economic, and cultural rights were adopted by the UN in 1966 by General Assembly in resolution 2000A (XX1), and were also ratified by Canada. This includes the right to work (Article 6), and the right to just and favourable conditions of work (Article 7). The upholding of these rights, however, is left to a weak system within the occupational structure of nursing.

Affirmative action and equality have become an area of intense debate that is sparked by neo-conservative orthodoxy in Canada. During the Harris government, affirmative action laws in Ontario were abolished in accordance with that government's political platform. Viewing social justice as part of collegiality helps examine processes within an occupational structure. I also discuss how discrimination prevents the development of collegial relationships, and how this leads to negative outcomes. Such a focus is necessary to illuminate how standards are set using collegiality, which is part of professionalism, is used within an occupational structure, without dealing with injustices that exist.

Staff nurses are a class within the hierarchy of the nursing profession, and the marker of colour is also a way to keep a group subordinate and disadvantaged. Equality of opportunity within occupational structures and within one's profession affects collegiality, professionalism, and the quality of life. Thus, the racial, social, and status hierarchy among nurses impacts on relationships in the work environment.

In order to understand the information provided by staff nurses about their work environment, I developed a model to examine staff nurse collegiality. Taken from Bess (1988), I use his three areas of structure, culture and behaviour. They are lenses through which I view the profession of nursing and collegiality. Differing from Bess, I focus on the structure of the profession as it helps us to understand the culture that produces the behaviour within the profession. Looking at behaviours only for answers will leave out the structural involvement within the work environment.

I have also examined a nursing leader's definition of collegiality to understand the interactions that occur among staff nurses (Styles 1982). In her attempt to explore professionalism and *professionhood* (p. 7), Styles provides the nurse with a list of collegial behaviours. Her argument is that the professionalism of nursing will be achieved only through the professionhood of its members. I contend that her view of collegiality does not adequately address the external and internal forces that contribute to the behaviours that occur among nurses. Further, she does not address the hierarchical structure within the profession, targeting behaviours, and the role of the staff nurse as it relates to her model of collegiality. As a starting point for this research, I do, however, discuss those items in Styles' work that make up collegial behaviours.

As stated earlier, nursing as a profession provides us with a case study where we can explore issues relating to occupational structures, women's work, as well as social justice and workplace abuse. The term "horizontal violence" (denoting hostility such as criticism, sabotage, undermining, infighting, scapegoating, and bickering, often propagated by nurses towards each other) is used here to describe dysfunctional nurse/nurse relationships.

It should be noted that racism within the profession and the workplace is another type of violence that takes place. Thus, institutionalized racism in nursing and the health care system cannot be ignored, as it is a question of social justice, and human rights; it is a form of racist oppression that usually gets lost in Canadian society.

The terms professional and collegial can be found in policies that govern the nursing profession. We see a complex relationship between organizational policy and organizational behaviours. While the stated objective of collegiality is about positive behaviours among nurses, voice must be given to the abuse, harassment, and racism that racialised nurses' experience within their work environment and their professional lives. Therefore, to understand nursing culture requires us to address an environment that includes issues of racism, and all other oppressions that lead to abuse and harassment, thus calling into question the claim that nursing is a caring profession.

In a given week, staff nurses interact with physicians, clergy, clinical nurse specialists, a nurse manager, a dietician, a psychologist, a social worker, a physiotherapist, a speech therapist, to name a few. In spite of their role, staff nurses are still on the low end of the decision-making ladder within their profession and in the hospital, and are not consulted when changes occur within the system. From the onset of this research, I knew that my "self" (Kirby and McKenna 1989, p. 20) was integral to the research and should not be discounted from it. Research from the margins is not research on people from the margins, but research by, for, and with them (p.28). Given my access to the environment and issue under investigation, I have decided to create knowledge rooted in the staff nurses' experiences, as well as my own experiences as a nurse manager.

This research began in 1994 and data collection continued until 2005. Using the snowball technique to involve subjects from over ten hospitals, a survey was designed to have input from staff nurses working in hospitals within Toronto. I viewed these nurses as the individuals who could interpret each other's interaction at work, and who would provide me with opinions about collegiality in their work environments. Interviews and focus groups provided the voices of yet another group of staff nurses who provided narrative experiences.

Information given on racism from one subject came in printed data from the individual's life story. The experiences, although personal, were given to me to share with others. This individual trusted that confidentiality would be maintained. She stated:

> There is a lot of injustice going on and it needs to be told when talking about staff nurses. Just tell it like it is. I can't wait to see your work if you really write what we tell you. (Interview, February 1997)[1]

Nursing internet list-serves provided a global context, as nurses' world wide 'talking' on the Internet brings a wider perspective. This was done in order to discover if the viewpoints provided by staff nurses in Toronto were similar or different to nurses working in other hospitals. Data was collected for four months seven days a week. This data was qualitative in nature and would assist in understanding the notion of collegiality among nurses in a global context.

The server, NURSENET provided a breakdown of the origin of the responses, listed by country. The majority of the participants were from North America, with the USA having 1,231 participants, and Canada coming in second with 367 participants. There were twenty-six other countries that participated in the discussion group.

The Organization of this Book

This book is organized into six chapters. Chapter one discusses dysfunctional nurse/nurse relationships; how privileged white women are oppressing other women especially racialised women, thereby denying them social justice. This chapter also discusses the positioning of racialised women within female dominated professions like nursing, and the fact that nursing research has mostly avoided dealing with this issue.

The "professional" nurse is discussed in this chapter in relationship to entry-level education, promotions, and workplace hierarchy. Included in this discussion is the make-up of the hospital community, and its effect on nursing culture. I address the work environment, professionalism, and collegiality with a focus on racism, and other abuses.

In chapter two I provide the reader with information on how the data was collected. I present the results of the research on the workings of the decision-making process, and the staff nurse role within the workplace hierarchy. I also explore 'the disconnect' between what the staff nurse group perceived as their role, and how the senior team of managers viewed the role of the staff nurse.

Chapter three speaks to the structures within the profession of nursing. The competing viewpoints of the four organizations, The College of Nurses of Ontario (CNO), the Ontario Hospital Association (OHA), the Registered Nurses Association of Ontario (RNAO) and the Ontario Nursing Association (ONA) occupy positions within the profession of nursing and can promote or block change that affects the staff nurse working within the hospital. The concept of collegiality and, by association, the understanding of "nursing structure," is central to understanding "the culture of nursing collegiality."

The production of culture within the nursing profession is explored in Chapter four. I review how nurse leaders within the RNAO, the CNO, and those within university networks form an "old girls" club. I show how this network dominates the direction and the vision of nursing, and helps set the career path for nurses whom they mentor.

Reviewing the behaviours of staff nurses and their lack of participation in the professional structures, I look at how these behaviours undermine their position. I suggest that this lack of involvement provides nursing leaders participating in the professional structures an important dimension of power over them.

This chapter discusses that nursing culture produces both conflict and collegiality; it has within it the value of caring that provides nurses at the bedside a reason for what they view as important to their role within the health care system. Nursing culture can also be understood through examining notions of the ideal nurse, the professional nurse, job promotions, and abuse and racism within the profession. In this chapter, I look at the wider social implications when dealing with the issue of racism within nursing.

Chapter five discusses behaviours within the third conceptualization of collegiality. Behaviour at the staff nurse level is related to the structure of the profession, and the culture of the profession. When discussing the issue of collegiality, staff nurses saw the negative and positive behaviours as associated with women working with each other. Understanding interactions described by staff nurses helps in the understanding of collegial behaviours that are threatened by the reporting of errors, complaints about other nurses' work habits, the rare encouraging of peers in risk-taking behaviour, and gossiping when other nurses have made errors. They also viewed helping and caring as important to staff nurses. Collegiality as Styles envisioned it, is not part of the everyday communication at the staff nurse level but is more in line with leadership values. In this chapter I look at how the largest group in nursing needs to come together—in the style of a silent majority—to challenge racism and abuse within the profession.

The final chapter is about how economic and social power is tied to understandings of collegiality, conflict behaviours, and inequality. Staff nurse groups in Canada can use advocacy to help "stir the cappuccino." Issues of social justice, including the injustices that staff nurses experience in the workplace and in the profession, must include analysis of inequities in promotions, in representations within their work environment, such as the Boards of ONA, RNAO and the CNO. As well, their voices need to be heard in government where health policy and changes in health delivery are made. Rather than going to the Human Rights Commission or the Courts, using advocacy, changes must first be made through the development of the 'self,' consciousness of the issues, and coming together as a group with an agenda for change.

The material[2] presented in this book hopes to focus the reader on the voices who provided insights and raises questions about a caring profession. The location of the staff nurse group within the health care system is like the location of women within society and affirmative action is needed for this group as well as racialised nurses within the profession. Empowering staff is more than words and those in power such as Members of Parliament, the Minister of Health, and the bureaucrats must address social justice issues that is currently part of the profession of nursing.

It is not those who are oppressed within the work environment who can change the system, the responsibility lies with the state, which has the power to makes the needed changes in occupational structures that disadvantage classes of workers. Staff nurses must, however, also come together as a group and have strategies to dissuade behaviours that would prevent a climate of collegiality from developing and encourage behaviours that make certain equity is part of the culture. It is through community interaction and advocacy that social relations can be addressed and changed.

Notes

1 Initials of participants are part of a system and not related to the individual.
2 Committees, organizational structures mentioned in this book may have disbanded or changed, however, they are used to present a picture of social and economic exclusion within the work environment.

Chapter One

The Cappuccino Principle:
The Racialising of the Work Environment

"Nursing, like a cappuccino—white on top, brown on the bottom—requires stirring up." Those words were the battle cry raised in a report submitted to the Canadian Race Relations Foundation (Hagey et al. 2005). The concept of professionalism includes altruism, accountability, autonomy (Freidson 1990) excellence, honour, integrity and respect. Nursing as a profession provides us with a case study where we can explore issues relating to social justice within a caring profession. In Canada, as in other societies, women still experience exploitation and oppression. Yet, not all women share a "common oppression." To understand the issues of difference, the profession of nursing, a female occupation, provides us with details of how social position provide some white women with affirmative action while racialised women are viewed as the "other." Within this caring profession, there is an unwillingness to acknowledge and distinguish white privilege and to realize that all women are not are equally oppressed. The women's movement in Canada as well as in nursing work life research have both failed to generate any in-depth analysis of how privileged women are in fact oppressing other women, thereby denying social justice for racialised women within female dominated professions like nursing. I use the term "racialised women" and not "women of colour" because colour includes white and the dominant society racialises the "other." Being different or 'the other' is *learned*, while being "Canadian" usually means being white and Anglo-Saxon. For the rest, we are all hyphenated Canadians, ethnic Canadians, or visible minorities courtesy of the Multiculturalism Acts of 1988, scholars, and the media. Rather than helping equalize cultures, multiculturalism helps separate groups with the false premise that everyone is accepted and given the same opportunities within an ideology of respect for diversity, but it failed, and fails, to acknowledge the dynamics of power and the entrenched privileges supporting employment and professional structures. Canada accepts more immigrants per capita than any other nation. It is estimated that close to 10% of the current adult population is made up of visible minorities, a number that is expected to double by 2016 (Institute On

Governance 2001). With this understanding we need to use this case study on collegiality to promote inclusiveness and equity within professions and in the workplace.

The concept of social justice is best understood as forming one part of the broader concept of justice. In general, social justice concerns the condition in which all members have the same basic rights, security, opportunities, obligations, and social benefits. It can also be understood by the differences in relationships, which I will explain by reference to features within social structures that exist in the profession of nursing.

To make these comparisons, I have drawn upon what is due to the individual within the work environment, and the treatment of racialised workers and white privilege. Social justice issues relating to our work environment are related to systemic social injustices and for rectification require advocacy activities committed to bringing about social change in current occupational structures combined with the addressing of the lack of opportunities that exist for some groups within the work environment. This means dealing with the distribution of power and the positions of decision-making as well as the reduction of fear and animosity among the work force. Analysing the structures helps us understand the cultural change that is needed to bring about equality and eliminating occupational injustices.

Racism and Abuse: How is this discussed in nursing?

Nursing is a dangerous profession and there are occupational health and safety implications (CBC News online 2006). Studies of workplace violence (Wagner 1992; Lusk 1992; ONA 2003) have revealed that mistreatment of nurses often occurs in places where it is least expected, such as in private homes, hospitals, and long-term care institutions. that arises out of patient assault (Cornerier 1990) is under reported and has legal implications. Dysfunctional nurse-nurse relationships (Taylor 2001) can also reach a point of physical abuse (Farrell 1997; Randle 2003). In an interview (1997) with me, a staff nurse reported that two female nurses pulled each other's hair and ripped clothing due to an argument over patient coverage. Dawson and Kehiayan (1988) associated the cause of hospital violence to the physical environment, high patient-staff ratios, inexperienced nurses, and poor interpersonal relationships. Graydon et al. (1992) investigated the personal and professional impact of verbal and physical abuse on nurses in Toronto. They found that at the time of the abuse, most nurses tried to resolve the problem. The most frequent type of abuse was verbal abuse. The nurses experienced abuse from the patient, their families, physicians, nursing peers, immediate supervisors, and other hospital personnel. Most of the subjects told a nurse colleague about the abuse, and almost all of the nurses told someone in the hospital about their abuse. At the time of the abuse, the victims found themselves experiencing increased heart rates, and their emotional reaction was anger.

In trying to understand beliefs and concerns about work safety and patient assaults, Poster (1996, 368) reviewed safety concerns, staff perform-ance, and legal issues and found that nurses who had been assaulted expe-rience a wide variety of symptoms such as anger, self-blame, and difficulty returning to the work setting. Poster stated that nurses around the world are victims of assault and that a significant difference in attitudes was found among nursing staff members who reported assaults. For most nurses, expe-riencing abuse did not make them feel less sure of themselves or less confi-dent in their abilities as a nurse. Some nurses commented that the public had unrealistic expectations of the health care system and as a result, people became abusive toward nurses.

Roberts (1991), and Ryan and Poster (1991) also reviewed nurse abuse in Canada. Roberts saw battered nurses as one more example of violence against women and found that nurses under-reported their responses to assault, felt blamed, and received little support from colleagues and management. Ryan and Poster reported that nurses in their study were uncertain about the legal and clinical issues of patient assault. Staff members who observed an assault also reported substantial stress. From an analysis of the data from workers' compensation boards over the past few years across the country for health care workers, the CBC (News online April 24, 2006) found these workers claimed five to twelve times more claims than any other worker. In the data there was no mention of racism in the workplace and days lost due to this abuse. The CBC, however, describes Canadian organizations as having a toxic workplace culture, and that Canadian workers are suffering because their employers have created dysfunctional workplaces.

The College of Nurses of Ontario (CNO) (1995, revised 1999) produced a programme on abuse which addressed the client but not one for nurses who were abused. The material focused on how nurses' behaviour could be abusive both verbally and physically, which they demonstrated in a video. This programme was intended to make nurses more aware of 'their'

11

behaviour and how 'they'—nurses should behave. In 2004, the CNO addressed the issue of nurse abuse on the part of patients as a practice guideline. A survey by the RNAO (Nursing Research 1992) stated that institutions themselves often tend to minimize the significance of physical assault on registered nurses and that physical safety contributes substantially to either overall job satisfaction or interest in leaving nursing. Since this survey, the RNAO (2002, Media Release 2005) continues working on women abuse but more so on women's issues in general—and not within the profession.

Race influences social interaction and positions whites in the centre of dominant discourses. Briefly, racism as a social construct refers to actions, intentional or unintentional, which foster ethnocentric standards, rules, and treatment of groups, people, and communities designated as different (Neugebauer 1995). Stereotypes, prejudices, individual discrimination, and systemic discrimination are mutually reinforcing. If there is systemic racism in a workplace, then chances are that individuals with power and authority in it are acting in ways that are adversely affecting "people of colour" (Das Gupta 1996, 13). As Foucault suggests:

> Disciplinary power is exercised through its invisibility; at the same time it imposes upon those whom it subjects a principle of visibility. In discipline, it is the subjects who have to be seen. Their visibility assures the hold of the power that is exercised over them. It is the fact of being constantly seen that maintains the disciplined individual in his subjection. (1977, 187)

Racism, therefore, is an ideology of supremacy propagated by the dominant culture where whites are in the centre of dominant discourse and occupy positions of authority and power. Racism, abuse, and harassment are part of the discourse of collegiality as race influences social interaction and group affiliation (Neugebauer 1995). Within the profession and the health care system, racism, abuse, and harassment are behaviours that are regarded as negative behaviours that are sanctioned against. Therefore, it is *un-collegial* to discriminate, however, racism, abuse, and harassment do occur within the profession and the health care system. The nature of collegiality within nursing must be a discussion of bureaucracy, power, and ethnocentric standards.

Farr details the work of Kathy Hardill, a member of Nurses For Social Responsibility in Toronto, who reviewed the topic of racism and nursing. The research showed a lack of Canadian material on this subject, while there was "a ton of literature from Britain and the United States on how racism affects nurses and how health care is delivered to non-whites in those countries" (Farr 1991, 9). Farr found that some nurses did not want to be identified in her article and they wondered whether the nursing profession was truly prepared to confront such a painful issue. She detailed the following from a staff nurse:

> Susan has observed other troubling patterns in the workplaces where she's been employed since graduating: a nurse with all the qualifications required for a particular job may find herself repeatedly turned down for promotion on the grounds of language skills. (1991, 10)

Most complaints about discrimination have arisen around the issue of language proficiency. Farr's interviewees felt that more formal study and exploration of the issues of racism and discrimination in nursing was necessary, and that it would be a pioneering and courageous move in Canada.

Building on the work of Head (1985), Das Gupta (1996, 2003) Calliste (1996, 2000, 2000a), Collins et al. (1999), and Hagey et al. (2005), we learn how systemic racism is organized in nursing and can develop an understanding of why these behaviours are related to the structures of the profession (Jacobs 2000, 2006).

In treating the topic of racism, Das Gupta (1996, 2004) provides a comprehensive description of how management practices create an environment for systemic racism. Her chapter regarding racism in nursing focuses mainly on Black nurses. Das Gupta views the everyday culture of racism as the exhibiting of behaviours such as targeting, scapegoating, excessive monitoring, marginalization, seeing solidarity as a threat, 'infantalization', blaming the victim, bias in work allocation, underemployment and denial of promotions, lack of accommodation, segregation of workers, tokenism, and co-optation and selective alliances (1996, 35-40). She describes scapegoating as a common experience whereby black nurses along with other nurses of colour are subjected to false accusations, blaming, and disciplining for unwanted events or actions in which they were not sole participants (1996, 77). She observes that the leadership in hospitals are predominately white (1996, 83), and that hospitals have a racist and sexist culture. She concludes that the form of harassment in hospitals is definitely "classic racial harassment" (1996, 87).

Although nursing in Canada does not wish to focus on racism and use concepts of diversity, or cultural competency to address discrimination, we know this social construction is built on stereotypes, prejudice, and the intersection of power. (Samuel 2005; Galabuzi 2006, and Visano 2006). Racism, unlike other abusive behaviours, leads to particular disadvantages, access to resources and mobility, and other opportunities pertaining to white privilege. To use words such as diversity, culture care, cultural competency, or multiculturalism prevents discussion of those who oppress, and looks at the "victim" or oppressed groups for the answer. Such language circumvents the fact that systemic racism is a problem that creates a toxic, poisoned work environment, where those who oppress are not always held accountable for their behaviours.

From time to time, the Ontario Nurses Association (ONA) tries to deal with racism, and pays for research on racism. The ONA's mainly white leadership addresses issues relating to social justice, and point to racism and discrimination in the workplace in its publication. For example, in *ONA News* of October 1994, it was reported that there was an increase in the number of grievances by staff nurses, and related several nurses' experiences in this regard. It was found that systemic racism and discrimination were almost impossible to prove through the ONA's grievance procedure, and also that the current system lacked expert arbitrators who could recognize discriminatory practices.

The ONA published another study on racism by Das Gupta (2002) in which she reported that 47% of the ONA membership had experienced the negative effects of racial discrimination in the workplace. The intention of ONA is to have a Human Rights and Equity Team with the goal being to achieve greater respect and dignity for nurses. Focusing on Human Rights and Equity in a publication and commissioning a study are positive actions, however, racialised nurses within ONA do not view the organization as a mouthpiece against racism in hospitals and within the profession. In 2005, Black nurses in a Toronto Local of the ONA expressed the view that the organisation itself practised racism when it came to dealing with conflict between white staff nurses and black staff nurses. Black nurses felt that the ONA took the part of white nurses against them. The collective charge by Black nurses that ONA has internal problems of racism stems from their perception of the union. In fact, these nurses have taken the ONA to the Human Rights Commission. They need the ONA to attend to racism as an everyday action, institutionally, just as it, and by extension, society deal with issues relating to gender and sexism.

The Registered Nurses Association of Ontario (RNAO) (1994) stated that in Canada, racism has been a largely very subtly taboo topic. They found that a significant number of nurses in Ontario to be "women of colour" and that nursing leadership did not represent nurses as a whole. Additionally, they noted barriers to higher education, and a lack of recognition for nursing education obtained from other countries. The RNAO (1994) stated that minority nurses have always been expendable, and are recruited in times of nursing shortage, and disposed of in times of nursing abundance. Yet in order to meet Canada's immigration criteria, nurses of colour were required to have qualifications exceeding those of white nurses.

Perhaps unaware of the colonial mentality that has endangered and subjugated peoples around the world (Battiste 2005), the nursing curriculum remains Euro-centred. Galabuzi (2006) suggested that access to professional employment was based on outmoded attitudes held by regulators and employers about the general competencies of immigrants from certain countries (133). He points out that these exclusions contribute to emotional and psychological stress of immigrants. Power elites would not label this learning environment as Euro-centric and racist but rather, would suggest that those coming to Canada lack Canadian experience and knowledge. They fail to view their gate-keeping role in the establishment of the curriculum (Galabuzi 2006). They also fail to acknowledge and account for hiring practices (Hagey and MacKay 2000) that include the unfairness of selecting certain protégées as behaviours that are not only unprofessional but contribute to inequality within professional and occupational structures. (Jacobs 2000)

The RNAO has policies regarding racism but like the ONA, the organisation has not been advancing the issues raised by the research (Das Gupta 2002) or by racialised nurses. Instead, the focus is on cultural competency (Beach and Price 2005), a concept that teaches health care workers to respond with empathy and respect to all races, ethnicities and classes by affirming their values and health care beliefs. Instead of applying anti-racist knowledge, this concept is being championed by those in positions of power. The issues of economic and social barriers must be addressed as equity issues relating to racism, not cultural diversity. Understanding diverse cultures has a tradition in the health care field but when it comes to put into effect true equity, there is a lack of "good will" on the part of those involved in setting standards of practice. Teaching staff nurses cultural competency or diversity will not root out systemic racism. Hagey et al. (2002) discussed how competencies have to be defended by racialised nurses even when they flagged the experience as racial discrimination, and were successful in actions against the hospital under the Ontario Human Rights Code.

Management can use competencies to perpetrate racism and harassment by citing failure to demonstrate cultural understandings to the satisfaction of management. It can be argued that cultural competency is a Euro-centric understanding of diverse cultures by placing groups without the intersection of class, ethnicity, generational variations, urban and rural differences. This monolithic view of culture allows misunderstandings to occur when providing service and care. It also allows management to rate staff performance as inadequate and undermining of administrative procedures. Thus, cultural competencies, rather than providing a way to decrease racism, can be viewed as tools that perpetuate racial and ethnic stereotypes within an increasingly discriminatory work environment.

The Hospital Anti-Racism Report (1994) developed a framework to implement anti-racist organizational change in hospitals and to prepare the provincial Ministry of Health (MoH) and the Ontario Hospital Association (OHA) for the assumption of a supportive role in the ongoing work of anti-racism organizational change. The Report addressed systemic racism and individual racism within the hospital sector, and described the criteria for a hospital's commitment to anti-racism. The published Report contained a framework for change that was understood by all board members, senior management, and staff of all hospital affiliates (OHA 1994). All of these organizations acknowledge that racism exists, however, there appears to be little evidence that anything is being done about the systematic discrimination that occurs in the health care system. In particular, there is a signal lack of minorities in management positions and in nursing education. Those who are in these positions had taken cases to the Human Rights Commission, or to their unions.

The lack of follow up by the Ontario Human Rights Commission on systemic racism in hospitals shows: 1) lack of leadership in the area or racism; 2) lack of monitoring; and 3) lack of commitment on the part of the

Commission in dealing with racism in hospitals. In two major cases in the 1990s, The Ontario Human Rights Commission dealt with racism in hospitals (Millelstaedt 1994) yet did not view these cases as the 'tip of the iceberg'.

The findings of the Hospital Anti-Racism Report did not change the nursing work environment. White privilege continued while the Harris government in Ontario discontinued Affirmative Action practices. Affirmative Action was important when it came to gender as it helped privileged white women to achieve their goals. These women, who were mothers, sisters, cousins, aunts, and friends of white privileged men, were afforded laws relating to Affirmative Action. This has not been the case when race was the issue. The message is that racialised individuals only need to be qualified, and once qualified, have an equal chance in attaining occupational goals, unlike women who needed affirmative action.

This situation begs the question: Are social barriers less for racialised individuals than for women who were usually white women? The answer to this question leads us to discuss the history of oppression in Canada. The ideological base of identity politics and *exclusivism* dates back to the period in Canadian history when European settlers and Aboriginal peoples first made contact with each other. Today, it is occupational structures that allow white privilege to enable inequality to flourish in the workplace. The situation has moved beyond seeing racial oppression as a media portrayal of minority groups, or the stereotypes that whites may have for racialised groups.

In a questionnaire "Are You a Racist?" (*Nursing Times*, April 1990), nurses were asked to complete the questionnaire to help explore how much they knew about racial discrimination in the workplace. Supporting ethnic and cultural diversity among nursing staff (Spicer et al. 1994) requires looking at similarities between providers and recipients. Spicer et al. viewed diversity as important and looked at the resources needed to support an ethnically and culturally diverse work environment (1994, 40).

Diversity training for hospital staff and the nursing profession was viewed as a method to cultivate a climate of tolerance. Occupational culture guides and interprets the tasks and social relations of work. Anti-racist knowledge instead of diversity training may have changed the culture that exists within the profession and in the work environment. The system is Euro-centric in training in spite of the diversity of the population. The orientation of newcomers is more about how the dominant groups view health, rather than the accumulative knowledge and cultural competencies that they bring with them to Canada.

The testing that occurs is very North American and is not familiar to immigrant nurses. There are other ways of evaluating skills and knowledge. Nurses with the same substantive knowledge can differ in their skill at solving abstract problems. Immigrant nurses may not have the Canadian classroom jargon but have experience that has been learned by working in hospitals prior to coming to Canada. Rather than blaming the foreign trained nurse for not passing exams or understanding the orientation process, the host country needs to understand how they test for competence or proficiency. It may be beneficial to have foreign trained nurses who work in the system orientate newcomers. They could use their experience and formal knowledge to explain the essential characteristic of nursing in Canada and address their questions. This discussion represents a Eurocentric way of educating "the other" (Jacobs 2006, 132-133). The profession and the workplace show concern about racism but do very little to combat everyday racist behaviour, systemic racism, and the mentoring of immigrant, racialised nurses.

The review of the above studies demonstrates the current understanding of racism within nursing. Traditionally, nursing has remained silent on the issues of racism. The Nursing Effectiveness, Utilization and Outcomes Research Unit, now called the Nursing Health Services Research Unit at the University of Toronto and McMaster University, reviews nursing work-life, evidence based standards, nurse/physician interaction, and gender. It has not, however, spent the dollars that they receive to address issues of racism within the profession. They want to ensure strong, visible nursing leadership at both the organizational and unit levels, and discuss magnet hospitals without one word relating to racialised nurses and their work life. In addition, through the Canadian Health Service Research Foundation (A Commitment to Nursing 2005), social science and sociology researchers, and nursing researchers have been provided research funding to create high-quality new knowledge on nursing issues that can be used by decision makers and managers.

Research Chairs funded for ten years since 2004 have not taken into account the disadvantages that racialised nurses experience in the system. Prior to receiving funding in 2004, the silence on racism in can be reviewed in their reports and books. The lack of Anti-racist discourse, and the lack of identifying racism only reaffirms for racialised nurses that the four research chairs in Toronto lack insight and understanding of the issues that racialised nurses face in the work environment and in the profession. Once again, the policies that they advance will be Euro-centric. The nursing knowledge network will not include racialised scholars and nurses who have much to contribute but are left out of the loop due to 'the old girls network.'

Perhaps since guns and violence have brought racism back to the surface in Toronto in 2006, we may see these researchers jump on the band-wagon and engage in studying racism in nursing. We know, however, that since the 1980s, racialised scholars such as Wilson Head (1985) and even the OHA (1994) have discussed racism in the hospital system. To date, major researchers in nursing who have received large research funds have not dealt in a substantial way with the issue of racism and nurse-to-nurse abuse.

In Canada, racism in nursing has been researched mostly by racialised scholars. Using much smaller grants these scholars have looked into the work lives of racialised nurses (e.g., Collins at el. 1999). Collins reported that an escalation in harassment took the following forms: a) perceived differential treatment; that is, denial of privileges granted to white nurses; b) problematizing the immigrant nurse of colour, and docu-menting the effects of the escalating conflict; c) labelling the nurse as aggressive, rebellious, unmanageable, etc., thus deterring support, polariz-ing the setting, and isolating the nurse; and d) full reprisal and punishment for a state of conflict perceived to be fuelled by management.

With the current restructuring of the health care system, the climate of working relations for nurses of colour is a chilly one. Participants' narra-tives in Collins et al.'s work provided data to support the perceived exis-tence of individual and systemic discriminatory practices. They gave accounts of positive experiences when they initially started work, but in the climate of restructuring of the health care system, discriminatory practices were exacerbated and predicated along in-group and out-group lines. Collins et al. recommended raising awareness and making racism more visible.

Minority voices within the nursing profession during this study also provided descriptions of encounters that they have experienced. Kirby and McKenna (1985) point out that too often the experts who do research have been well trained in patterns of thinking that are counter-productive to an anti-racist project, and that they explain and justify a world many of them are really interested in changing. For Kirby and McKenna, research and knowledge are used as instruments of power that impose form and order for the purpose of control, thus maintaining oppressive relations. Information is interpreted and organized in such a way that the views of a small group of people are presented as objective knowledge (1989, 15). In keeping with their book *Methods From The Margins* (1989), the research presented here reflects and analyses the social context of collegiality from the staff nurses' perspective—the perception of their interactions, as these nurses are on the margins of the production of knowledge within their profession.

Within a profession and/or organization, when issues such as racism occur, the organization forfeits the loyalty of those experiencing racism. Institutional racism is the systematic reproduction of inequality within fundamental structures and processes.

Normative roles and rules and ideologies and their everyday applications operate to oppress and devalue the "other," the non-whites. In addition, minority communities speak a different language, practice different customs, and share different worldviews. Race as a social construct based on specific historical and geographic contexts of the experiences of individuals, is viewed from the standpoint of the individual experience with many interpretations regarding the social organization of a society.

We cannot address work environments without focusing on racism and other abuses. Racial discrimination (Hagey et al. 2005) exits but is not discussed as a top priority for a healthy work environment. Institutionalized racism in nursing and the health care system cannot be ignored, as it is a question of social justice. There is a generalized fear of backlash around the raising of issues concerning racial discrimination. This fear is warranted because of the culture of silence and the lack of knowledge about the nature of racial domination. Dominant messages reiterate: "everyone is tired of hearing about racism" and the feeling is that everyone is bending over backwards to try to be politically correct. Hagey et al. (2005) reported that they identified four types of "set-up:"

- Targeting individuals
- Top-down orchestration
- Recruiting peers
- Pre-emptive or reactive documentation.

They point to the following counter-strategies that can be implemented for potential effectiveness in addressing each type of set-up:

- Identifying supporters
- Gaining influence
- Recruiting powerful allies
- Strategically using documents.

The targeted racialised nurses are set up in such a way that focus is shifted from a clinical or administrative problem onto the racialised nurse, who then becomes the problem. As Essed (1991) defined it, racism has the effect of problematization. The rules of the set-up strategy make the nurse who complains about this state of affairs a target so that accountability and transparency are impeded. Benefits accrue to the nurses and administrators who collaborate in the set-up. Racialised nurses are drawn into set-up activities with the effect of deflecting attention from the racially based strategy. This process makes accountability for set-up practices highly improbable, especially in light of the potential for being targeted for complaining about the problem in this strategic system.

The strain on racialised workers around the reporting of harassing behaviours and in speaking up against discrimination is a dilemma that needs to be recognised as it helps us to accept their construction of silence in order to defend their economic life and their energy. Asserting one's rights looses its appeal when one is faced with backlash and termination. In order for collegial relationships to really occur, we need a true understanding of workplace social justice wherein each worker has the right to participate equally in the process. Such changes are needed to acknowledge white privilege and to establish that social justice for staff nurses is not accomplished by 'professionalising' their behaviours. Instead, they need to be provided with influence and access to shared decision making about organizational change. Thus, the issue would be seen as a human right issue and would not require the services of high-priced lawyers, paid with tax dollars, to uphold management's side in the dispute.

Hospitals would then not act as fiefdoms, for they are owned by the taxpayers. Rather than discounting human rights complaints, hospitals need to represent their staff who have been ill treated and humiliated, intervening on her or his behalf, and mediate an outcome and change in their organizational culture (CRRF 2005).

It is clear that what happens in the work environment affects not only the worker but also the family, as work and family are linked. Duxbury and Higgins (2003) researched work-life conflict and states that it is asso-

21

ciated with increased absenteeism and substandard organizational perform-ance. They point to a lack of supportive culture in Canadian organizations, work overload, and employees not being seen as contributors. The study points to a workplace culture that is toxic, even without dealing with harass-ment and abuse. This research helps us understand the spill over that occurs outside of the work environment as well as how home-life affects work-life. As most staff nurses are female and have care- giving responsibilities at home, the stress they experience in their work environment makes them both physically and psychosocially more susceptible to stress related injuries.

Nursing – other areas of research

Work environments are not stand-alone entities but are created out of vari-ous decisions that come to the environment from organizational structures that govern it. The nursing profession is a fairly new professional category, having recently been transformed from the status of a semi-profession (Jacobs 2006). It is still, however, at the margins of power within the health care system, and within this marginalized group is yet another group which has even less power. This group consists of the racialised nurses who work within the profession.

In the restructuring of the nursing profession, primary nursing replaced team nursing in order to give staff nurses and patients a form of continuity of care, and to give the staff nurse some level of autonomy. This strategy gives the staff nurse accountability for care outcomes without the necessary resources, and leads to blame and horizontal violence. The term "horizontal violence" (denoting hostility such as criticism, sabotage, under-mining, infighting, scapegoating, and bickering, often propagated by nurses towards each other) is used here to describe the way in which some hospi-tals pit nurse against nurse by establishing such roles as "primary nursing" that isolate some nurses (see Rounds 1993).

Following the assumption that nurses are typically and traditionally non-assertive, Kilkus (1990) views self-assertion as the tool by which nurses, coming from a long history of subordination and identification with passivity can make their voices heard. He viewed assertiveness as one of the tools that can be used to construct a new model of caring based on strength, honesty, and respect. Research on nurses in Alberta (Mitchell 1971) found that nurses were not interested in professional development activities such as collegial relationships and that further education was a personal and not a professional goal. Vance (1977) reported that nurses identified major disadvantages of belonging to a predominantly female profession as including problems of self-image, lack of career commitment, lack of power coupled with political knowledge, limited perspectives, and the impact of family and personal responsibilities. This is perhaps due to a tight influential circle from which others are excluded, and thus feel disenfranchised, and invisible.

To interact with each other and to create a system of support, nurses will need to create a very large circle from the multiple circles that currently exist (Kilkus 1990, 135). They need to develop support systems, networks, and coalitions of like-minded colleagues who join together for mutual benefits (Vance 1982). The support systems can range from mentors, sponsors, and guides, to peers and friends. This would very likely have an outcome of the reduction of conflict. Another suggestion for improvement that is advanced by Baumgart and Larsen (1988) is that all nurses have a role in providing support, opportunity for career advancement, and more importantly, assisting with cultural change. Support, respect, and assertiveness are viewed as behaviours needed within the nursing profession, and are linked to either professional or collegial behaviour. These ideas, starting in the 1970s, are still significant in improving nurse-nurse relationships, and reducing horizontal violence.

Shared governance for nursing is viewed as creating a new organization (Porter-O'Grady 1991). "Shared governance," the terminology used when hospitals put nurses, such as Nurse Managers, in charge of budgeting and staffing, is to Rounds (1993) yet another bogus concept. The hospital gives this governance entity a budget within which they cannot possibly work. Nurses then end up fighting among themselves about work time.

Earlier studies (e.g., Murray 1988a, 1988b) have identified the real needs of nurses, and have called for long-term strategies to address career problems. Porter-O'Grady views the nursing license as an agreement between the nurse and society and suggests that professional practice and properly shared governance models are based on clear definitions of accountability. In a real shared governance model, role ambiguity is not acceptable at any level, thus quality assurance becomes a clinical process and not a management activity. As such, the peer review becomes an ongoing obligation of every member of the nursing staff (1984, 699). Another term, "career ladders," is hospital language for merit increases. Rounds reported, "If you are a good girl and rat on another nurse, your supervisor will move you one rung up the clinical ladder. The hospital asks for team-work, but what really happens is that they reward one team member at the expense of another" (1993, 38). It is important to consider the work envi-ronment in terms of job satisfaction, the organizational culture and the rela-tionship of staff nurses and nurse leaders. This provides a framework where job satisfaction can be understood, not only as a numerical assessment, but also as a climate that produces collegial or conflictual behaviours within the organization.

All these concepts are, however, issues targeted to benefit patient care through creating an environment whereby nursing staff provide input and are accountable. When they change strategic plans, hospital administra-tors and their Boards need to include front-line nurses from the very begin-ning, rather than leaving them to follow their manager's lead. This manager usually has very little influence and is not viewed as a change agent. "Collegiality" is one way of examining behaviours in a work environment to ascertain if true inclusions by Nurse Managers occur, if horizontal violence occurs, and whether or not the Human Rights Code and 'social justice for all' are parts of the work environment. Behaviours point to the type of culture within the work environment wherein relationships are hier-archical and conflictual, rather than collegial and inclusive.

Understanding Collegiality

Research on collegial behaviour has been limited. The formal definition of collegiality is "the sharing of authority among colleagues." This authority is vested equally in each of a given number of colleagues. The terms "colle-gial" and "collaboration" are used interchangeably and can be linked to communication. Collegiality is an attitude about professional behaviour and relationships that leads to collaboration and respect for the other. Collaboration among members of the group becomes one of the elements of collegiality. Many authors (e.g., Jordan 1983; Boyle 1984; McMahon 1990; Coeling and Cukr 1997) describe only the expected behaviours of collaboration and the need for such behaviours to exist within the profession.

In these formulations collegiality is more about categories of behav-iours that construct what is deemed as a "collegial" nurse. The collabora-tion model is based on the belief that it is necessary to create and maintain a learning climate, something that is viewed as an essential ingredient for the development and maintenance of quality care. Greiner for one (1972) describes collaboration as an organizational state characterized by spontaneity and problem-solving across functional areas. The process of collaboration is actualized as each person accepts the other's goal, and the desired outcomes of each participant are obtained (Schmidt 1974). Often, collaborative communication results in the determination that perceptions were inaccurate and that no real conflict actually exists. Such communication promotes an opportunity for groups to strengthen themselves through valuing each member's contributions, and by replacing competitions and criticism with concrete, supportive communication aimed at co-operative action, acknowledgment, and validation (Hurst and Keenan, n. d.).

Hurst and Keenan note that colleagues provide feedback in the form of constructive criticism and praise. They also posit that a collaborative climate requires and fosters a shift from communication focused on judgements and changing people, to communication that is encouraging, supporting, acknowledging, and validating (n. d., 27).

Colleagues and collegiality (Gagnon 1991) are about learning from each other, sharing issues of the nurse's experience, sharing educational resources, and strengthening relationships. In Gagnon's view, the way to begin is to build on the shared experiences of colleagues. It is clear, however, that status and role conflicts involve tensions generated by structural controls within the institution (Roth 1982). Roth represents collegiality in nursing by comparing it to an all-pro football game wherein senior administrators control the players, as do physicians, and by default, the hospital Board. The specialties of nursing practice can be equated with the individual football teams (Roth 1985). To successfully resolve these problems, nursing would need to clear up individual differences in the pursuit of unity, with responsibility for creating an environment that promotes collegial relationships lying with those nurses in management (Nolan 1976, 43).

Social meaning of nursing collegiality is constructed through the everyday interactions that occur on the units in which nurses interact with each other. In any review of the concept of collegiality, the issue of conflict arises. One area of an ongoing conflict is the process that emerges in interactions between individuals competing for scarce resources. Stress and burnout are other areas that relate to collegiality, in that interpersonal relations affect the level of stress that occurs within the work environment. Among nurses, I argue, oppressed group behaviour manifests itself in the tendency for subordinate groups to direct their frustration toward co-workers rather than toward those who oppress them. This is exemplified by and inclusive of administrators. Conflictual behaviour is manifested as gossip, errors in medication, the reporting of these errors, and blaming behaviours. Although nurses could handle errors and reporting in a collegial manner, they seldom discuss this behaviour.

Bess' study of collegial behaviour in universities (1988) discussed three components of such behaviour: culture, structure, and process of behaving. He describes them thus:

> ...three distinct components, two of which are relatively static, the other dynamic. This first is culture (or normative framework); the second, decision-making structure; and the third the process of behaving, which is constrained by the first two. (1988)

For Bess, culture, structure, and behaviour make up the major components within decision-making, and he looked at how decisions were due to a normative framework.

In *Images of Organization*, Gareth Morgan (1986) examines organizations and explores their development through structure, culture, and systems that contribute to the theory and practices of organizational analysis. Culture is also a part of the interactions that reference groups can provide to the individual. This changes as the meanings attached to symbols are changed, and as the environment both within and external to the group changes. Therefore, an approach that considers structure and culture provides for a framework for the comprehension of staff nurse collegiality within hospitals.

As individuals interact over time, structures organize their actions in relation to one another. Structures can be seen as organizations or as social patterns, and include decision-making structures within organizations or professional groups. The term signifies the organizational life of a group and/or certain practices that are a part of the organization, such as governing boards. Decision-making can be found in formal and informal gatherings, and decisions for most of the organizations discussed in this book are made from the top down. Individuals in decision-making structures are engaged in the process of creating organizationally desired behavioural outcomes, and so are also regulating behaviours of their workforce.

The identification of social structures needs to be done by considering the complex relationships that occur between them. Using a lens that identifies power and authority, each part of the system must be analysed as to how it affects the staff nurse group as well as the other parts of a given professional structure. In this book, four major organizations, the Registered Nurses Association of Ontario (RNAO), the Ontario Nurses Association (ONA), the College of Nurses of Ontario (CNO), and the Ontario Hospital Association (OHA) are discussed in their relationship to the nursing profession. Along with them, I review the role of the Ministry of Health (MoH) and the Joint Policy and Planning Committee (JPPC). Since the MoH provides the health care system with funding, and through the JPPC, is involved with planning within the hospital system, it impacts the nursing profession through both their funding of hospitals, as well as through funding of nursing projects. Hospitals are included as part of the structure of the profession as they employ most nurses. We see that hospitals are medical bureaucracies whose goals are to conduct business as efficiently as possible. Therefore, the structure of the profession is also discussed as it relates to bureaucracy where decisions are made that affect the staff nurse group. As a group of employees, staff nurses provide their views through the ONA. Staff nurses also interact on units/wards with each other. These sub-units also influence the behaviours that occur among the staff nurses on each unit. The research indicates that units have individual subcultures and produce conflict and collegial behaviours that can be unique to a unit. For this study, however, it is important to focus on the structures that impinge on staff nurses from a distance, and the actions that affect their work-life. I do pay attention, however, to the dynamics of unit subcultures and the effect unit culture has on behaviours.

The organisational culture is created through activities classified and validated by communication and sanctions. These experiences become interpretive practices, and are the currency and criteria of the institutionalized experience (Neugebauer 1995). Culture also becomes the lens through which social worlds are refracted. Thus the self is constructed as a conscious product mediated within cultures of subjectivity (Visano 1987). Staff nurses are intimately linked through interaction to their group and the culture of the group, both at the unit level as well as at the larger professional level. Self is constructed in interaction, and that interaction is influenced by the larger group in the organisational context, and by society, in

27

the larger context. Goffman (1959), describes the concept of collegiality, stating that non-collegial persons are those

> who present the same routine to the same kind of audience but who do not participate together, as teammates do, at the same time and place before the same particular audience. Colleagues, as it is said, share a community of fate. In having to put on the same kind of performance, they come to know each other's difficulties and points of view; whatever their tongues, they come to speak the same social language. And while colleagues who compete for audiences may keep some strategic secrets from one another, they cannot very well hide from one another certain things that they hide from the audience. The front that is maintained before others need not be maintained among themselves; relaxation becomes possible. (Goffman 1959, 180)

Goffman's theory of front and back stage provides us with a way of understanding collegiality. He purports that the stage where collegial behaviour takes place is in the area of the "front stage," which is, in our case, the observable behaviours of the staff nurses. The line dividing front and back stage is everywhere in society. Our behaviour when we do not have an audience is back stage behaviour. Front stage collegiality can be viewed as the interaction that takes place when other individuals, such as peers, managers, or patients, are there as observers and/or the participants. Back stage collegiality occurs whenever the individual is no longer observed but still behaves in a collegial manner. An example of this would be when a nurse answers a call bell for another nurse. Sharing information or gossiping when not under observation can be interpreted as back stage behaviours. Of course, organizational culture also produces front stage and back stage collegiality.

We can view collegial behaviour as occurring in both focused gatherings and unfocused gatherings. Focused gatherings in nursing occur when the patient care teams meets, or in committee meetings where there is a preordained structure of expected conduct. Unfocused gatherings in nursing occur when emergencies in patient care take place, such as for example, a cardiac arrest. Both focused and unfocused gatherings provide individuals with the opportunity to learn norms and values of the group, or of the individuals within their professional group. These behaviours provide some level of collegiality in a relationship between the individuals sharing the information.

The culture of the profession is discussed in this book as it relates to the norms and values passed down since Florence Nightingale and the interactions that have occurred between nurses over time. The voices of staff nurses provided most of the data for interpreting nursing culture. When reviewing the culture of nursing within Ontario, I note that as nursing leadership changes within the structure of nursing, it also affects the culture of the ideal, professional nurse.

Within the profession of nursing, a value is placed on professionalism. The professional nurse is discussed in this book as it relates to entry-level education, promotions, and hierarchy. Included in my discussion is the make up of the hospital community, and its effect on nursing culture. As noted above, organizational cultures also include subcultures that occur on individual units. Subcultures have cultural forms that carry ideological messages from which come collective understandings and patterns of behaviour that pertain to the group. When the staff nurses on a unit transmit the unit's ideology to the newcomers, they play a part in the socialization of these newcomers. Therefore, the culture of collegiality can differ from unit to unit. It is, however, the voices of staff nurses that best describe nursing culture as they have experienced it.

The three areas of structure, culture, and behaviour are lenses through which I view the profession of nursing and collegiality. Focusing on the structure of the profession helps us to understand the culture that produces the behaviour within the profession. I see structure as providing for culture, while Bess views the culture as providing for structural decision-making. By linking the understanding of "micro" social actions with a "macro" understanding of organizations, we can account for social life without neglecting the structural settings in which these actions occur. Thus, social order in the workplace setting is constituted by different, if not conflicting, discourses (Neugebauer 1995).

Given that staff nurses experience serious alienation from their organizations, their work, and each other (Hansen 1995, 11), there is no useful model for the understanding of collegiality in an organizational setting that has been developed to guide administrators in enhancing collegiality between nurses and other health care providers. Hansen depicts collegiality as work group cohesion, job involvement, and substantive exchange in the give and take among co-workers of valued work-related, social, and personal benefits. She describes collegiality as reflecting the exchange of resources, ideas, skills, needs, concerns, and personal support. These are more likely to occur where nurses believe they genuinely participate in work-related decisions, both in terms of institutional policy-making, and personal work activities (1995, 18).

Hansen views collegiality as a unique condition among members of a definable formally organized professional work group, which is characterized by non-hierarchical relations, group cohesiveness, interpersonal exchanges and collaboration. Within the nursing academic setting, collegiality is valued as a requirement for promotion and tenure. It includes the willingness to serve on committees, to perform work necessary to departmental operations, a demonstrated willingness to provide guidance and help colleagues, and to respect the ideas of others (Balsmeyer et al. 1996, 265).

Another view of collegiality comes from Styles, a nursing leader, who uses her formulation to examine the interactions that occur among staff nurses. In her attempt to explore professionalism and professionhood, Styles provides the nurse with a list of collegial behaviours (1982, 7). Her argument is that the professionalism of nursing will be achieved only through the professionhood of its members. Within this framework, she describes the characteristics of collegiality as an attitude about individual nurse-to-nurse relationships. According to Styles, collegiality is "the sharing of responsibility and authority with colleagues and is based on ultimacy [sic] and leads to respect" (1982, 143).

A concern with this model is that it is advanced from a nurse leader who holds an elite position within the profession. I contend that Styles' view of collegiality does not adequately address the external and internal forces that contribute to the behaviours that occur among nurses. Further, she does not address the hierarchical structure of the profession, nor the targeting behaviours, racism, and other abusive behaviours within the profession. There is a lack of attention to the role of the staff nurse as it relates to her model of collegiality. As a starting point for researching work-life behaviours, I did, however, adopt Style's items that make up collegial behaviours. I did so with the caution that her view of collegiality leaves out the staff nurse.

Since the 1980s, staff nurses informed me of harassment and abuse, sexism, and racism as well as feelings that management was passing down to them the cutbacks that were occurring within the hospital. I also became aware of the pervasiveness of inequality within the nursing profession while Styles was looking into collegiality. Staff nurses were angry and complained about the hospital environment, their peers, the physicians, and especially nursing management as subjecting them to bullying. In the nursing profession (Randle 2003) bullying has effects on self-esteem, an aspect that Styles did not address. Many of the observed behaviours pointed to gossip, complaints, and blaming. In addition, when discussing collegiality Styles did not address racism, an issue that has become an overt factor within the hospital system in Toronto. This resulted in racialised nurses bringing cases against two hospitals to the Ontario Human Rights Commission. The first case had the support of the labour movement rather than the ONA, which did little to push this landmark case. (OHA Anti-Racism Task Force 1996)

Hospital culture will be discussed as it relates to staff nurse collegiality. This work environment has been changed by political decisions embedded in the constant shifting of power as one government falls and another takes power. This history of change in policies is a concern, not only for the delivery of health care but also affects nurses' work environment. The change in nursing work because of decisions made by wave upon wave of political ideologies uses the delivery of care as a battlefield in the struggle between private and public funding for our health care system. Hospitals have grown in size and complexity to the extent that decision makers within most hospitals are members of the Board of Trustees, Chiefs of Services who are physicians, Hospital Administrators, and sometimes Nursing Management. Clinical Managers have been replaced with Operational Managers with little or no clinical experience in patient care. In addition to this, there are many types of individuals providing bedside care to patients, some of whom are professional and some others who are non-professional, such as Personal Care Assistants. On the question of providing patient care, most hospitals function at the level of "a team": There are registered nurses, registered practical nurses, health care aids, and sitters, all of whom provide patient care.

During the last two decades, nurses have seen groups of other professionals come into hospitals and take over functions that they once performed, or that were not available within the health care field. The manner in which these individuals communicate and interact with each other is also an aspect of collegiality within the hospital work environment. The stated focus is often 'Quality Care', yet in praxis, it is on the financial strategies designed to ensure that the organization achieves operational success.

The work environment for nurses was one wherein female nurses were subordinated to male dominance, both by virtue of being female in a patriarchal society, and by being seen as assistants to the male-dominated medical profession. Stripped of its historical, religious elements of loving care and self-sacrificing duty, nursing is revealed to be a female ghetto of cheap labour. Nowadays, nursing finds itself as a scientific profession that is still highly labour intensive. The major influences for nurses today are the rapid proliferation of biomedical technology, and the changes in communication systems. The value of caring is still important to staff nurses, however, and they make up the largest group of nurses within the profession.

In order to connect with earlier perceptions and research regarding nurses, I use the work of Hughes (1958) who described the nurse in the following manner:

> In the drama of the treatment of the ill and the injured, the nurse is in the center of the action in every scene. Never the prima donna, she is the stalwart character who must always be ready to pick up a missed cue. She keeps the action moving. Hence she knows the play better than anyone else. In the days of crises and of so much change in the organization of health institutions and services, she can make a greater contribution to the understanding of this great drama then can any of the other characters to any of the spectators. (1958, 351)

Hughes' view of the nurse in the center of the action best describes the staff nurses within the hospital system, yet the system does not acknowledge their unique role in terms of positions on Board committees. Staff nurses occupy an interesting position within the health care system and can be viewed as "the nurse closest to the patient". These staff nurses co-ordinate the treatment and care of the patient assigned to them, and are closest to the patient in the day-to-day activity in any hospital. They also provide most of the care and treatment for their patients. In a given week, staff nurses might also have to interact with physicians, clergy, clinical nurse specialists, a nurse manager, a dietician, a psychologist, a social worker, a physiothera-

32

pist, and a speech therapist, just to name just a few. These positions are needed in the organization but the role of the staff nurse is one that as Hughes points out, "is the center of the action", and must be viewed as different from all other roles. In spite of this, staff nurses are still on the low end of the decision-making ladder within their profession, and within the hospital. It is interesting to note that they are not consulted when changes occur within the system.

It was mentioned earlier that the development of nursing as a profession has been dominated by the influence of patriarchy. Male doctors and administrators created the institutions where female nurses work, and although women have become 'players' in areas of medicine and adminis-tration 'the game' is still influenced by the history of its roots. Nightingale's vision was under male dominance as doctors and superintendents viewed nurses as no more than cheap labour. Today, hospitals exercise control over the work nurses perform, even though nurses are licensed by their profes-sion, and use nursing labour when and how they wish. Due to the caring (and therefore feminized) nature of nursing, however, the work is not valued, and nursing is viewed as an example of household work that has been shifted to industry. This leads to a premise of this research that staff nurses can be viewed as an oppressed group because they lack control and power within the institution, just as women lack power within society's industrial complex.

The Staff Nurse Role

Travelbee as early as 1966 describes the nurse as follows:

> ...an individual who has been irrevocably and profoundly changed as a result of her specialized knowledge and educa-tion. She has learned a body of scientific knowledge and has the ability to use it, has developed new skills; but more important, she has been confronted with the vulnerability of the human being in a way that an adolescent of young adult entering another occupational field has not. The most profound changes are brought about by exposure to illness, suffering and death, in that these experiences are irrevocably removed from the status of comfortable abstractions, becoming instead profound realities. (44)

The initial studies concerning nursing roles were conducted in the 1960s (Corwin 1961; Corwin and Taves 1962; Travelbee 1966; Harrington and Theis 1968; Kramer 1968, 1969). This work provided a way of looking at nurses that grew out of research by people such as Peplau (1952) who defines nursing as "a significant, therapeutic, interpersonal process, an educative instrument, a maturing force, that aims to promote forward movement of personality in the direction of creative, constructive, productive, personal and community living" (1952, 16). Travelbee (1971) views the purpose of nursing in this way: "to assist an individual, family, or community to prevent or cope with the experience of illness and suffering and, if necessary, to find meaning in these experiences" (1971, 16). Both Travelbee and Peplau are interested in the potential for the nurse to understand the helping process and therefore focus on the interpersonal processes. They view the nurse as an individual who possesses a body of specialized knowledge and the ability to use it for the purpose of assisting other human beings. Travelbee also states that a nurse practices only in circumscribed areas that have been defined (1971, 44). The nurse is perceived as educated, experienced, and as working predominantly within hospitals.

It is clear that in these early studies, researchers did not look into the areas of collegiality, nor did they use the term "professional nurse". Discussions centred on issues around the semi-professional status of the work, authority, and the role of the nurse (e.g., Hughes et. al. 1958; Ross 1961; Suryamani 1989). During this period of research, nurses were aspiring to professional status but had not been granted it by the public, their employers, and researchers. We can contend that in part, nursing was seen as women's work and professions were being reserved for men.

As stated earlier, rituals within nursing help provide meaning to the role. Words, actions, objects, gestures, and relationships are important to ritual performance (Wolf 1988). The study of nursing rituals demonstrated that nurses valued the procedures and customs associated with an undertaking in their work. There were patient rituals, therapeutic nursing rituals, and occupational nursing rituals. Rituals have been described as valueless and are often condemned or seen as cherished beliefs in need of abandonment (1988, 59). There are, for example, rituals around giving medications, taking care of the dead, and admitting a patient. Nurses learn rituals during their training, and on the job from senior nurses (Ross 1961). The study of rituals within nursing (e.g., Wolf 1988) uses sociological concepts in the understanding of how nurses construct their rituals by placing everyday events and making distinctions between the sacred and the profane.

Role socialization studies (Coudert et al. 1994) have examined graduating student nurse role conception and changes that occurred during a concentrated clinical preceptorial (which is much like an internship that occurs for the medical profession). Coudert et al. found that staff nurses influence the role orientation of neophyte nurses, provide effective work-centred role models. They also conclude that when exposed to clinically experienced role models, nursing role conceptions are changed or altered through learning and work experiences. The researchers also found that the faculty may tend to be more idealistic than their staff nurse colleagues. The study supported the lack of congruity between faculty and staff nurse perceptions of the nurse's role (1994). Taves and Corwin (1963) state that there is an important relationship between one's occupation, her or his occupational self-conception, and her/his total identity. Therefore, I argue that staff nurses get their identity from their peers rather than their leaders, such as the nursing faculty.

In researching staff nurse collegiality, the information obtained showed that the requirements of formal training in nursing, and the discussions around the definition of who is a professional have been significant in causing conflict among staff nurses. The quest for professionalism through higher education contributes to the polarization around issues of who is a better-trained nurse, and so provides for an area of conflict within the staff nurse group. Another element of conflict that staff nurses encounter is the constraints that bureaucracies have on professionalism. Professionally, when they discover an error, nurses are expected to report a colleague. This behaviour is encouraged in order to enhance the public's safety when mistakes occur within a hospital. All of these ingredients are impediments to collegiality.

Although nursing is considered mainly women's work, rather than focusing on feminist issues around medical dominance and white male administrators, this book explores how staff nurses interact with each other within the hospital environment. The book also explores how this work environment supports conflictual behaviours, making it a toxic work environment for many of the front-line workers. I discuss how the women in power within this work environment use white privilege to enhance their role. Like their white male counterparts, white elite women in nursing have a network to enhance their work-life, and maintain their positions of power.

In times of scarcity, minorities become vulnerable, and as structural changes occur, they are the first to be laid-off by the "knowledge elites" who define "professionalism" (Glazer and Moynihan 1975). Thus, institutional barriers and practices around meritocracy and equal opportunities are understood within the social structures and forces within the profession of nursing and the health care system. We have discussed the fact that nursing literature is limited in this area. We have also noted that the production of racism within the framework of collegiality creates conflicting subjective positions, especially when it comes to racist discourses. Nevertheless, collegiality in an urban area such as Toronto cannot be discussed without encountering the issues of harassment, abuse, and racism, as there are power relations, conflicts over resources, and ethnocentric ideas that produce institutional barriers for racialised nurses within the profession. If I failed to raise these issues within the context of collegiality, I would not be accurate in formulating the issues around nursing work life.

We cannot look at nursing work life without accounting for men who work in this occupation. Men in nursing comprise a small percentage of professional nurses in North America (Squires 1995). These male nurses fare as well, if not better than their female colleagues, and are over-represented in administrative positions (Williams 1995). It would appear that several assumptions exist around men in nursing. The two most common inferences and stereotypes heard about men in nursing are (1) linkages to homosexuality, and (2) that these men who choose nursing as an occupation really wanted to be physicians but were unable to achieve this.

These stereotypes are a form of abuse, and yet men in nursing seldom report abuse or harassment. In this book, I did not make gender an issue when discussing the responses provided by staff nurses. There was no significant difference in the level of position, wages, and seniority that men in nursing were given compared with their female counterparts. In terms of the staff nurse positions, union contracts determine the job descriptions but there is a differential between male and female nurses when it comes to promotions. Like their female counterparts in nursing, I found them to be concerned with the same issues, such as the quality of care that patients receive, and the lack of time to deliver that care (concerns related by A.R., staff nurse [1996], A.J. [1995], V.D. [1997]). As the following nurse stated:

> I am a nurse, not a male nurse. If I am standing in front of someone of talking to someone on the phone, it is perfectly

obvious that I am male. How many times when a women physician introduces herself to a patient as "Hi, I'm your female doctor!" No, its "I'm your doctor." Same thing, I am a nurse that is male not a male that is a nurse. (G.G. 1995)

G.G. provides the basic response that I received from male nurses when discussing their gender and collegiality. I note, however, that men bring with them internalized values that allow them to voice their concerns, and not be submissive and subservient (R.H. 1997). It must also be noted that the work environment for male nurses has advantages for them. This is manifest in the fact that while they constitute a relatively small percentage of the nursing profession, male nurses do make up a disproportionate number of management positions that provide them with power and financial gain.

For racialised male nurses, the work environment is similar to that of racialised female nurses as these men are often in staff nurse positions, while their white male counterparts climb the ladder to make up the disproportionate number in management. Are male nurses more collegial, or do they have communication skills that lead to connecting with male senior administrators? These questions cannot be analysed since individual narratives did not enter into these areas of discussion. It is worth emphasising, however, that men in the work environment did express that they were not abused and were often addressed as "doctor." Racialised male nurses also informed me that they were addressed as "doctor."

Occupationally linked sex role stereotypes appear to be stronger for nursing than for other professions. When lay people are asked to evaluate the role of staff nurses in health care, they usually rely on information acquired from the mass media. Yet nurses are in constant contact with patients in their homes, in hospitals and clinics, as they provide the care and treatment for their clients.

Physicians, individually and collectively, have perpetuated the myth in public that nursing was subordinate to medicine, and should remain in that position for the good of the public. The public at large still perceives nurses as doing what physicians tell them to do when they are admitted to hospitals. Therefore, maintaining stereotypes and public misinformation about nurses reinforces the notion that physicians are superior, both in knowledge and skill, and that nurses are the physician's handmaidens.

Both the ONA and the RNAO have dealt with shared myths and images from the mass media. Both organizations have used education as a tool to inform the public about misunderstanding the nature of nursing and nursing care, and to raise the profile of nurses today. Although I deal with some of these issues, they are discussed in a limited sense only as they relate to staff nurse collegiality.

In this book, I provide details about the relationship between staff nurses who work in acute care settings, using the concept of collegiality. Most of the encounters (Goffman 1963) that occur within the staff nurse group take place as part of the day-to-day activities that occur in the context of their roles as nurses. Staff nurses provided narratives that have been included when discussing the data from the survey. By providing the voices of staff nurses, the understanding of the behaviours that make up collegiality can be viewed through their eyes. In understanding what behaviours are important to the staff nurse, collegiality can be constructed at this level of nursing. When constructed from the voices of the staff nurse group, we glean insight into the injustice that the nurses feel they have experienced, and their perceptions of being in a toxic work environment.

We know, however, that work environments differ. They grow out of complex human relationships that are constantly shifting, and are controlled by many different competing agendas. What is clear from the research is that women, whose work as caregivers is devalued in society, find the same thinking reflected within the health care system. A major area of concern that perpetuates this thinking is the fact that staff nurses, although central to the care of patients, are not represented at the Board level, while physicians have their voices heard. Through their exclusion, we can see how they determine the way they are viewed within the hospital structure and the health care system, and it helps us to understand the construction of nursing care and the role of women's work.

We need to include the role racialised women play in nursing, and explore the feelings they have of being exploited as cheap labour. This is especially important when they are employed as Personal Support Workers (PSWs), replacing the work that was done, first, by Registered Nurses (RN), and then by Registered Practical Nurses (RPN). As the cost of employing one category of nurses increased, work was downloaded to the less-trained category. Today, the PSW who has the least training works in long-term care facilities as well as in acute care and in the community.

Although government, hospitals, and the public state that registered nurses are needed and valued in the system, through organizational actions and workplace practices, the RN is replaced with the RPN, and then with the PSW. This is done without consulting the staff nurse as to how these role and work changes impact on the work environment within the hospital. These actions send a message to the staff nurse that her/his work is devalued within this type of decision-making process. Administrators who make decisions around nursing consider budgets and are concerned with trying to cut costs. PSWs who have minimal training are attractive to administrators, as they are the lowest-paid caregivers. As wages for the RN increases, hospitals make decisions, not on what they do but on how much it costs to hire an RN. Rather than viewing a bed bath as an assessment, they view it as a bath that anyone with minimal training can do. This type of thinking looks at the task and not at the process of holistic care that occurs during a bath.

Most PSWs come from racialised groups, and are segregated at the bottom of the health care hierarchy. They do care-giving work, are not licensed, and are not nurses. The patient, on the other hand, does not know the difference between a PSW and an RN and will view a woman in uniform giving care as a nurse. An important question to raise is: "Why are these racialised women are not given the chance to become nurses when we are short of nurses in Ontario?"

When discussing staff nurse collegiality, the constraints of present economic policies, "downsizing," hospital management culture, and the decision-making system within the health care system are examined. Once again, I would like to emphasize that the voices heard in this study provide the data and the understanding of their experiences of hospital life. Thus, it may appear that I have not provided a forum for the administrative viewpoint but this has been deliberate and is not an oversight. It is not intended that the issues be presented in a balanced way, with each side given the same space. The intention is to look for the expressions and insights of those whose voices are seldom heard within the nursing profession, the hospital and health care system. Clearly, the elites in nursing have a forum through government funding of their research, and it is through this professional structure that one comprehends the culture within which staff nurses interact with each other. In addition, we can see the implications of this interaction for our healthcare work environment.

One needs to ask the question: If workers are unhappy, how do they provide the best possible patient care? This book tries to address several questions by discussing the construction of collegiality that I feel is central to the ongoing debate of nursing care, nursing work life, social justice, and human rights, as well as the location of nursing as a profession within the health care system. In looking into the interactions of nursing, I hope to stir this cup of cappuccino and provide my colleagues with issues of social and economic justice and ideas about where change needs to take place.

Chapter Two

Why Study Collegiality?

During the 1990s, the RNAO promoted professionalism, and within professionalism, was also the expectation of collegiality (Styles 1982). When in committee meetings, Nurse Managers discussed how nursing behaviour could change to reflect a more professional image and develop research-based practice in our hospitals. Part of professional behaviour is the component of "collegiality" which is idealized, and used as a standard to evaluate nurses. I asked staff nurses to discuss these questions, and I also reviewed my own experiences in this regard. I wished to understand if staff nurses felt that they behaved in a collegial manner, or if behaviour between nurses was rather more 'conflictual'.

I chose to survey nurses across Toronto who worked in hospitals that provide acute care. This focus, I hoped, would bring a measure of objectivity to the investigation about the reality of collegiality within a larger group. I wanted to know the prevalence of staff nurses' respect for each other, or any other of the 'ideal type' items that were discussed by Styles (1982). Utilizing a component of quantitative analysis in this study is intended in part to counteract any subjectivity (by which I mean overt subjective *over*-bias) that I would have had as a participant-observer, inasmuch as I lived inside the world of the subjects being researched. Yet, since group percentages provide in aggregate form the views of the group on an attitude or issue, the members within the group provide the perceptions or feelings around their work-world. Given that nursing work is viewed as "woman's work", and as undervalued by cultural ideologies constructed by the profession, and within gender and institutional hierarchies, then we can understand collegiality and lines of communication. We can see that it is not just an issue of gender relations but is a function of the structural expressions of the oppressive practices perpetrated on women.

As mentioned earlier, a review of the nursing literature reveals that staff nurses' interaction with each other has not received a great deal of attention. I chose staff nurses as the primary focus because staff nurses represented the largest group within nursing and had the highest level of interaction with others—doctors, administrators, and patients—in hospitals as compared to all nurses in general. The other reason for this choice was that I found that nurse leaders expected collegiality to be a part of nursing performance, and used words such as "professionalism" when discussing nursing work. This is done without rather than asking the recipients of this standard, the staff nurse, what they considered collegial or professional behaviour.

The notion of collegiality is a complex issue that, when observed, would provide insight and knowledge of how interaction between staff nurses occurred on an ongoing basis. Applying nurse leader Styles' understanding of this concept to the intelligence in this arena may denote a privileged status to behaviours that may not be deserving of such status. My argument is that nurse leaders provide nursing theories to strengthen notions of professionalism that in turn empower the management class.

Given the bias toward women's work, collegiality could be used as a standard to discipline staff nurses rather than empower them. Therefore, we can question the concept of collegiality within the notion of professionalism. These questions beg examination: Was collegiality an important issue for the staff nurse in order for her/him to function within the eight- or twelve-hour shift within a hospital? For whom was the notion of collegiality important within nursing? Were nurses collegial in their behaviour to each other? These kinds of questions help us to look beyond Styles' claims, and tell what the staff nurse feels about her/his role and identity within nursing as it relates to gender, society, and ethnicity.

Kirby and McKenna's notion of "research from the margins" is about taking control of the information that we present which has been presented on our behalf in the past (1989, 18). According to Kirby and McKenna:

> The margins refer to the context in which those who suffer injustice, inequality and exploitation live their lives. People find themselves on the margins not only in terms of resources. Knowledge production is also organized so that the views of a small group of people are presented as objective, as "The Truth." The majority of people are excluded from participating as either producers or participants in the creation of knowledge. (1989, 18)

Staff nurses are at the margins of nursing; knowledge production is organized by a small group of white women situated in positions of power. Some reside in universities where nursing is taught, some in the halls of health ministries, while others are in hospital management. The construction of knowledge is also the construction of nursing identity. It is critical to note that this 'knowledge-making' is done within a Euro-centric framework, and provides a distorted identity. As occurs in the capitalist market, economics plays a role in the production of knowledge, with the State as a powerful presence allowing these differences to occur. More work needs to be done as to why government research dollars flow to a small group of elite nurses who help formulate the issues around nursing work-life.

An important aspect of this discussion is what the majority—the staff nurse group, views as peer group interaction and collegiality within their work-life. With this kind of information, the nurses and their settings are not reduced to categories of dependent and independent variables but are analyzed in the context of the setting in which they interact. As we construct meaning through a process in which individuals interpret behaviour and assign meaning, the staff nurse group becomes the reference group. Thus, the quantitative data provided by the survey measured a value of the individual respondent within a larger group of respondents. This information enables a deeper understanding of the issues from what I will call "a reference group's point of view" as defined by the respondents themselves.

The next step was to take the survey to the staff nurses working in Toronto. I canvassed staff nurses who agreed to provide the survey to other registered staff nurses in their hospitals. In total, thirteen registered nurses working in ten hospitals were approached. They agreed to participate in the survey research and to contact individuals within their peer group to participate in completing the survey. These nurses approached registered nurses working in hospitals within Toronto, and thus provided a research link with registered nurses (RN) with whom I had no prior contact.

Nurses within the institution where I worked and who were from various clinical environments also participated in the survey. Within my institution, I contacted a staff nurse who acted as the contact person, thus distancing me from collecting the completed surveys. Four hundred self-administered surveys were handed out over a six-month period through a "snowball" approach to hospitals within Toronto. A total of 142 surveys were completed and returned to me by staff nurses from ten different hospitals. Participation was anonymous as I did not go through management or involve them in any way in order to provide the staff nurse with confidentiality, and the promise that management would not review their answers.[1]

Data collection took place between 1994 and 1997, and participant observation was ongoing throughout this period until 2005. During the time of this research, my position was that of a nurse manager, and later on as a casual staff nurse. In order to be a part of the staff nurse group, I spent time with nurses at the staff nurse level who worked in different hospitals and at their homes, interacting with them on topics of work and the health care industry, and interviewing them, or arranging a focus group. At these times, their friends, who were also staff nurses, would drop in and join the discussion.

It seemed clear that to research the relations between staff nurses, it was essential to present the experiences of the individuals in their natural environment. Throughout this period, the knowledge that I used was an interpretive paradigm that allows the individuals the ability to know themselves and understand the others. The other part was to understand who was attaching meaning to the interaction. The survey as a research tool helped me feel objective during my fieldwork where I had been making observations and in which I was a participant. The conflict between objectivity and subjectivity is ameliorated when a holistic approach is used that is sensitive to multiple constructed realities and their concomitant biases. This strategy would emphasize subjective meaning among the several versions of interpretive methodology studies. The emphasis on experience served to understand not just collegiality but nursing work and attitudes toward the work environment.

An interactionist perspective directs the problem for empirical investigation (Visano 1987), and it was also the understanding that I, the researcher, was starting from my own experience, and required more information to guide this research. Collegiality had been discussed by those in the nursing literature, but not from the perspective of the major group of nurses such as the staff nurse. In my observations, staff nurses working in hospitals have not participated as equal partners in the creation of knowledge, or policies. As explained, my aim was for the staff nurse group to participate in and provide an understanding of staff nurse interaction and collegiality so that their interpretations of actions, the meanings they attribute to concepts, and the analytic meanings they assigned to situations in which they participate could then be heard. Interviews with staff nurses disclosed information about their activities, looking backward at the conditions that shaped their actions as subjects (Denzin 1989). The framework consists of the concepts and their interconnection within the specific social context within which the study is focused.

The participant observation approach arises from the concerns that the researcher, within the interactionist framework, grasps at first-hand the social world in question (Visano 1987). This methodology provides an inside look at social life for those individuals who are involved in the data gathering process. Participant observation combines various methods of gathering data, such as surveys, personal accounts/narratives, life histories, document analysis, and direct observation. This allows for as full an account as possible of how individuals make sense of their experiences (Kirby and McKenna 1989, 76). Ethnographic participant observers attempt to understand some group or community with the suspension of the researcher's preconceived ideas that he or she may have had of the group. As a nurse manager at the time of this study, I tried to make sense of my role, my relationships, and the work environment.

In making an account of collective behaviours in a descriptive manner, I was involved in sharing the norms, values, beliefs, and socialization of the respondents involved through direct contact and a long-standing participation with individuals who were part of the research. The reflection on events by the researcher is not one of total immersion but rather that of sharing information of the experience of the social world first-hand, and observing interactions in the workplace. This closeness to the subjects provided an understanding of the language and expression of central meanings.

Through participant observation, a researcher becomes acquainted with a peoples' *weltanschauung*, or worldview (Visano 1987), and this type of fieldwork permits the researcher to provide intimate accounts of the social processes and personal experiences. As a nurse working within a hospital doing research on a topic that I was in contact with on a daily basis, I did not have to play a role, as that of another non-nurse researcher coming into the environment. My participation was one of complete participation because I was both in the world of my subjects, and also was myself 'a subject' as I documented my experiences. My main focus, however, was to understand the meaning of the world of staff nurse collegiality, which was a level away from my daily interactions. This meant that I would have to discuss several topics with staff nurses, such as the concepts of respect, sharing, help, gossip, and blame. The meaning of the behaviour viewed became a major task. It required a meeting with staff nurses from other institutions and those from my own institution, in order to seek their understanding and analysis of relationships, communications, and culture of the work environment. As a research topic, "Work" also had to include the experiences that had occurred in my own work world. My own feelings around role autonomy, racism, and abuse would have to be understood within the methodological framework of the research, and the experiences that were documented.

As I gathered information, the rapport that we developed made me a sounding board for the participants. The "grapevine" — the informal network of communication in the hospital—provided a rich source of information. I noticed that most of the time nurses' knowledge of my research activities did not deter them from speaking openly. They continued to feel comfortable discussing issues of importance to them, inclusive of their negative feelings towards management. There were moments when I forgot my research, and became part of the group.

What became apparent was that I identified with the role of the staff nurse within the system. It became an important task for me to examine my feelings. Was I writing because of my feelings as a student nurse, a staff nurse, and now a manager? This was not complete participation, as I was not working as a staff nurse, and I was not in any disguise with the subjects involved. Being aware of and attending to moments of transference, that can surface and inhibit effectiveness of the research also provided a tool for understanding nursing work. If any unresolved feelings, attitudes, and wishes were brought into present exchanges, they could have distorted the task of getting to know the meaning from the other's point of view.

I left full time acute care hospital work in 1997, and worked as a casual staff nurse until 2005. This break in full-time nursing allowed some time for reflection when dealing with different aspects of nursing work. Over ten years of data collection and research points to 'disconnect' that is occurring between the staff nurse and her\his work as well as her\his profession. The politics of the health care system denies the place that the staff nurse has within that system by discarding the role of the Clinical Nurse Manager, who not only relates to the work of the staff nurse but had also been a staff nurse. Today, nurses are managed by non-nurses or by nurses with little 'bedside' experience, and more 'book' experience. It was important to examine if there were any implications that this management change has for patient care. It was equally necessary to examine whether those in charge of our health care system took into account the implications of a toxic work environment that exists in hospitals.

During the time of my research, the work environment in Toronto hospitals was negatively affected by the Government of Ontario, and continues to be destabilized by constant changes by the government of the day. Staff nurses work in an environment that is constantly changing and where the Ministry of Health announces cutbacks from time to time. In spite of nursing shortages, job insecurity became, and is still a problem.

During lunches in the cafeteria, I would sit with different groups of hospital staff and was thus privy to discussions about job issues. One group consisted of staff nurses, a second was nurses in management, and a third was a mixed group of staff, physicians, and non-nursing management. These groups usually did not eat together but instead, sat in specific areas apart from each other in the cafeteria. During these periods, I carried out informal interviews through conversations. Many individuals who were newcomers to the institution also provided information on issues concerning their nursing professors, the institutions where they had worked, and how they had been treated as student nurses.

My management role permitted strategic access to information in the form of written documents, as a routine part of the work-world. These came as letters from administration, letters of complaint from patients, and from physicians. I decided to use this information as background qualitative data while providing anonymity as an adjunct to my formalized and informal questions.

During most of the data collection phase, I did not enter into interaction with staff nurses when issues arose between them. This was not hard to do as I was not a staff nurse at the time, and was usually not noticed by the involved parties. At times, I heard casual conversations that took place between staff nurses who were either sitting or standing near me, and who were well aware of my presence nearby. It is also important to note that I did not actively control interactions that had particular bearing on my research; even in informal groups, I allowed the communication to be led to subjects such as hockey, or baseball, and many times did not touch on the subject of inter-hospital issues. It would have been easy to usurp the topic and point it to the staff interaction, as "something" was always happening. I felt that open encounters were more important than contrived communications, and I wanted to make sense of what I heard, and grasp the properties of the subject's meanings of the situation or interaction that they were discussing. Many of the conversations led to negative comments towards senior administrators, physicians, and nurse administrators.

Collective knowledge was obtained through nursing journals, especially from the College of Nurses of Ontario's *Communiqué* that carried letters and articles from and about nurses. Analysis of these letters and articles provided information about issues of abuse, mistakes that nurses make at work, about behaviour that is deemed unprofessional, and about standards for nurses. I sought to understand how beliefs were articulated, and what was important for the CNO.

Although to a limited extent, the CNO's newsletter, *Communiqué* provided discourse at the institutional level about the professional structure of nursing. Most of the discipline notices in the *Communiqué* concerned the staff nurse who worked at the bedside with certain behaviours being viewed as "unprofessional" and with the names of individuals published in the newsletter. Another source of information came and the cases that staff nurses brought to ONA against their employer. This research was structured in a manner to provide a voice for the staff nurse around behaviours, while the information in the *Communiqué* assisted in understanding the structure and culture of the profession as discussed by the professional body.

I undertook interviews in order to obtain life histories. Due to the constraints of the time on the part of the registered nurses and shift work, interviews were difficult to obtain. A total of eleven individuals, both male and female, were contacted. This approach was the most frustrating and difficult to achieve, as I wanted an even number of males and females in my sample of interviewees. I went to individuals' homes, and if acceptable to the interviewee, would tape the interview. Some respondents wanted to tape their life histories without me. In those instances, I provided them with the questions that I had prepared as a format for them to tape their stories.

While there were certain questions that I wanted to cover with each interview, I allowed for variations to occur when the respondent wished to express an issue that was her or his concern. I used all of the skill I had as a psychiatric nurse, relying on interviewing techniques that I had acquired in this field. Verification of nurses' experiences and feelings was not an issue because the individuals were providing me with their perceptions and feelings around being a staff nurse within a hospital system. I relied on other participants and survey data to provide an overall system for cross-checking the recorded stories.

As reality is socially constructed, it is in constant change. My research had started prior to the restructuring of Toronto hospitals, and as I write this book, the process of hospital restructuring is still occurring. The fear of job loss was a major issue, and the shortage of staff was another large concern. Issues of racism and lack of respect and abuse became a more open topic of discussion with racialised nurses. These issues were discussed even at the management level in nursing. As the research progressed, I found that my own life history needed to be included in the overall research. I too was making sense of the world in which I worked, and the research was an answer to my own questions concerning nursing interaction. Having ongoing contact with nurses from several institutions allowed me to check my impressions, and guard against subjective conclusions. I concluded that research that is experientially grounded provides a richer database, with greater detail, and adheres to an interpretive paradigm with a preference for grounded theory (Glaser and Strauss 1967). I also realised that neither the life of an individual, nor the history of a society can be understood without understanding both.

I found another group of nurses on three different websites on the internet who were discussing issues around communication, role autonomy, "eating their young," the presence of males in nursing, and abuse in nursing. Attending to these conversations provided me with more information at the global level. I explained my project to users of these sites and was able to obtain information from them. Although they were informed that I was studying collegial behaviour among nurses, this did not stop the interaction and communication on the nursing sites. Here were nurses talking to each other about what happened to them in their workplace, the responses they received from the chat group, and their own responses. I found myself more of an observer at these sites, a "lurker," and did not participate in a direct manner. When I put out the question on collegiality, I did not receive many responses, however, I did receive references of work done in the area.

In general, staff nurses hoped that this study would help articulate their feelings about their role, and how they related, not only with each other but also with management, patients, and physicians. Lack of support for my research from my senior nursing management was an issue for me that created stress. In fact, a senior nursing administrator found a copy of my survey, and accused me of causing conflict among physicians.[2] She informed me that she had not given me consent to circulate the survey in the hospital. The statements were made without my input and even though

49

I informed her that I had not circulated any surveys, she put her objections in writing. I did not, however, allow this nurse administrator to deter me, and responded with a letter to the president explaining my research and method; the matter was then dropped at the organizational level.

In retrospect, the behaviour of senior nursing management was not only abusive and threatening, but helped point me to research areas of racism and abuse within nursing. It also shone a light on the role the president and senior hospital administration play in determining how decisions are made, and how hospital culture affects nurse-nurse collegiality.

It is important that the researcher is accountable in some way in the research. It also helps the researcher to focus on the topic, and to formulate the question. As I began looking at the content of my experiences, the focus of the question became clearer, and helped me understand and incorporate data from my own experiences as a nurse. Perhaps the question of collegiality in nursing disturbed me and caused a concern when I observed that the majority of behaviour outside of formal committees had not been one of collegial behaviour within the nursing division. I had seen and experienced both horizontal and vertical abuse such as undermining, criticism, sabotage, and scapegoating. Nurses who were viewed as not being a part of the established 'group think' were set-up by others to fail. Reporting behaviour was part of nursing hospital culture. Yet, nursing leaders discussed collegiality as part of professional behaviour that needed to occur both at their level and at the staff nurse level. To the observer, it showed a leadership that did not 'walk the talk' but was interested in establishing a profession on the backs of the staff nurse. I recognised that the survey questions were important to me, as I discussed collegiality and what nursing leaders were communicating about nursing behaviour. It meant that they needed to be constructed in such a way that the responses would shed light on the discussion on nursing collegiality.

The first time I examined my own perspectives and biases as a nurse took place in a group discussion with my former classmates who had come to Alberta for a class reunion. We discussed the issue of why we had chosen the field of nursing, and why some had left the field of nursing. I remembered thinking of nursing as an inexpensive way of getting an education as nursing students were given a monthly stipend from the government during their training. Student nurses who were trained in Hospital Schools of Nursing had a bond with each other, as they felt verbally harassed as a group by staff nurses, physicians. As a group that trained together for three years, we were supportive of each other.

As a psychiatric nurse, I recognised that observation is a part of the profession that is taken for granted. Nurses observe their patients for depression and other signs and symptoms that occur both on a verbal and non-verbal level. When my interest in nursing behaviour began, I would discuss the issues that came up at group meetings, both at a formal and informal level. The informal discussions with staff nurses and nurses in management began prior to my interest in the subject of nurse collegiality. In 1990, I found myself observing and participating in discussions around professional behaviour in nursing. Communication was about nurses acting in a professional manner, and so I made observational notes and collected data on how I was treated within the management group that was made up mainly of white women. On reviewing these notes, I became aware that targeting had occurred, and that as a racialised woman, I was constantly challenged, while the white nurse managers were allowed latitude with the same behaviours.

Some of these white female managers met outside of work for bridge, and other social events; they also communicated in the hallways about new ideas or changes that they wanted to see occur within the organization. This behaviour helped to form an "in-group", even within management. Another action that occurred was the de-skilling that took place from these white nurse managers. Racialised nurse managers were constantly told they did not do a "good job", even when it was not their jurisdiction. Some nurses referred to them as "the Fancy ladies" who "felt that the nursing profession belonged to them." As immigrant patterns change and we become a more racialised society, this tension between what racialised nurses called "the white elite women" in nursing, and their racialised counterparts has serious consequences for the profession and patient care. It highlights the need to implement the Section 5(2) of the Ontario Human Rights Code (ORHC 2005) which states that:

> All employees have a right to freedom from harassment in the workplace by the employer, employer's agent, or by another employee because of, among other grounds, race, colour, ancestry, place of origin, ethnic origin, citizenship and creed. This right to be free from harassment includes the workplace but also the "extended workplace", *i.e.* events that occur outside of the physical workplace or regular work hours but which have implications for the workplace such as

business trips, company parties or other company related functions.

Unfortunately, Section 5(2) is not viewed by white nurse leaders as a code by which they must abide, nor do they acknowledge that the behaviours they engage in contravenes CNO standards. It is clear, however, that the Human Rights Code needs to be applied to workplace culture and employee rights.

At times researchers discuss social phenomena as only that which is observed, however, social phenomena is also experienced. Observation enables inter-subjectivity and critical reflection to become clear to the observer. On the other hand, inter-subjectivity and critical reflection throughout an analysis ensures that we are able to hear and affirm the words and experiences of the research participants, and at the same time, are able to critically reflect on the structures that influence our day-to-day work lives. Although not all institutions are identical in every situation, there are similarities that can be understood through observational data.

The data for this book consisted of everyday interactions on units, informal interactions, and formal committee meetings. At the same time, I was also maintaining a paper trail on activities that were occurring in my work life. My employers had been terminating racialised, experienced managers, stating that they did not have credentials to be managers. As a racialised manager, I had an M.A. and a background in management, and was at the thesis stages of my Ph.D. The senior administrators who were all white did not meet this level of formal education but did not view my achievements as adding to the position I held as a manager in the area of Mental Health. The question arose as to "What did a sociology degree have to contribute to nursing?"

I found that I was excluded from information, was monitored more than other white managers, was criticized and undermined. One very new nursing director in her first week as my director informed me that I had been working "too long" at the hospital, and that I should be looking at another institution for work. This woman took it upon herself to start a hidden file on me. She also asked physicians and my staff to give their feedback on my work, and their judgements on how I managed the unit. The very physicians whom she interviewed related the situation to me.

The troubling aspect of this racist behaviour is that the same individual is now employed in the education of nurses. This fact-finding did not occur with the other managers who also happened to be white, and were under the same director. If this style of selection is how she decides who is "right for the position," then my concern is how would racialised students fare under her tutelage? My work was constantly supervised and the Vice President of Patient Services gave me a five-page letter disciplinary letter. Even though this individual lacked management experience, did not have a degree in nursing, was in her first position as a manager, she was promoted in a very short space of time and thus, felt empowered to harass me. As if it were her right, she constantly spoke down to me, and refused to have me receive a 'retention package', something that she gave to all of her white nurse managers and to herself.

Considering this to be racism, I challenged both the letter, and the retention package. This job-related stress, and racism were areas that I was researching and now was experiencing in nursing. The stress that I experienced was extreme and caused me to visit the emergency department with rapid heartbeats, and high blood pressure. During these years I found it difficult to compose arguments for this research, however, it helped me to understand the world of racialised nurses within the health care system, where white women get promoted, mentored, and assume positions of power, while racialised women with similar or superior education and skills are bypassed. Other racialised and ethnic-minority managers expressed the same job related stress, with some reporting depression, and other mental health symptoms. They spoke of de-skilling and verbal abuse. I labelled all of these behaviours as racialised abuse, and white privilege within a toxic work environment.

As stated before, the cafeteria and the hallways within the institution provided me with back-stage information and behaviour. I was able to observe first-hand how co-managers treated staff. There was unfairness, and a lack of respect for the views of staff nurses. I found some managers speaking poorly about staff nurses as a group as being expendable, and replacing them with cheaper labour such as health care aids. One manager spoke about her staff during a committee meeting as "pigs eating from a trough" when she saw them taking some food from a tray. This statement was uncalled for, yet her superior did not reprimand her.

The lack of respect and the elitism of the managerial group have serious implications within the health care system. Speaking with managers from other hospitals, I found out that due to cutbacks, this type of behaviour was also occurring in other hospitals. It is interesting to note that at times when staff nurse positions were being cut, management positions were increased through clinical and education positions. Committees were top-down, and decisions were not made as co-equals. Senior Nurse Managers and senior hospital administrators would constantly seek ways of changing the system in order to be within the provided budget. At the same time, however, they spent monies for their own retention packages, and those of managers whom they deemed to be important to them. These Senior Nurse Managers also brought in new management techniques using consultants to enhance quality care without any attempt to have the staff nurse group buy-into the process.

This points to a 'disconnect' between what the staff nurse group perceived and how the senior team of managers viewed the role of the staff nurse. The feelings that I had as a manager toward senior nursing management and administration were mixed. I went from anger, to distrust, to tension, and back to anger and distrust. This hospital was the location where I had received my training, and I found myself torn between the past and the present. Reading the paper trail that I had kept over the last six years of my employment, I became aware of the abuse, and concluded that a group of women educated at the masters level in nursing, behaved, not as colleagues but as privileged white women used to dominating others.

Nursing departments produce relationship structures through organizational charts. Organizational charts determine where decisions are made and where the staff nurse role is within the hierarchy. Committees were still loaded with managers and staff nurses who did not have a real voice. As a staff nurse working in psychiatry, I was expected to speak out for our patients and be a part of the team. With this research, I wanted to provide a voice for the staff nurses on the topic of collegiality, and to allow racialised managers to be heard. I knew and was told that many nurses did not speak up because "they needed their job" in an environment of nursing surplus in the early 1990s, and with rampant downsizing. There was also the feeling that as an oppressed group they did not feel that their voices would be heard. Today, with a shortage in nursing, staff nurses do not have the same fears, yet, they do not speak out against abuse or racism.

Beginning in October 1997, I participated in a study on racism and nurses, and found that my experiences were not much different from that of other racialised women. This process helped raise my understanding of the dysfunctional nurse-nurse relationship (Taylor 2001). The distance from the hospital environment did not lessen the experiences I heard from other staff

54

nurses regarding the lack of respect from management, the lack of communication, and the lack of teamwork. Nurses had a scarce resource—namely, the time to do all the work required by administration. The ability to do their work became difficult, and brought with it behaviours that will be described later.

Through my conceptual baggage I realized that I had come to believe that there is a group of senior white nurses who want power and control of the profession within Ontario. These women meet when at university and form bonds, and then hire each other and maintain a network in order to maximize their power and status. There are other nurse leaders, however, who are inclusive, even though they may be in the minority. Unless racism in nursing is discussed openly by the profession, the current group that excludes racialised colleagues will continue their behaviour. The treatment that I and many other racialised women experience will be brought to light in this research.[3]

The goal of this study was not to defend the concepts of collegiality as described by Styles but to provide an exploratory account of the perceptions and the values of the staff nurses, and the relationships that occurred among them. Rather than assuming as Styles described from her standpoint, that collegiality was perceived by nurses, the symbolic interaction paradigm postulates that individuals in everyday life create reality.

Notes

[1] I treated all information and individuals contacted with respect and safeguarded the subjects' right to confidentiality. In this research, the choice of going to a hospital's Ethics Committee for approval provided me with the dilemma of having an opening to subjects with the approval of administration or going to the nurses directly. The dilemma when involved with two equally unsatisfactory alternatives provides for choice where one party would be upset. In the first instance, it would mean that the research met standards of the hospital involved but could make subjects distrust the researcher. In the second instance, allowing the subjects to give out the surveys did not allow the hospital's committee to approve the research, and this restricted the pool of subjects who could have been available for the research. Having heard staff nurses complain about research projects that came to them via administrative channels, I had second thoughts of using management as a way of reaching subjects. I wanted participation to be voluntary, with the subjects having full knowledge of the questions raised, all the while reconciling competing interests. My decision was to go to the staff

nurses through their peers. Names and initials assigned to the participants have been changed to protect the identity of the individuals involved.

2   Maintaining records in a safe place is an additional aspect of confidentiality. I made sure that I did not leave documents written by individuals in my car or in areas where others could view them.

3   The colleges and universities also lack women of colour as educators. This is another area for research in Ontario.

Chapter Three

The Structure of Collegiality:
A Case Study of Nursing in Ontario

Analysing the complex institutional relationships that occur among the various nursing spheres of influence, where interactions among the leadership are in the form of decision-making, information networks, rewards, strategic alliances, and conflict, can identify social structures. In this chapter, I describe important structural relations between nurse leaders, hospital administrators, government, and the larger structures within which these relations are embedded.

Since most employed Registered Nurses work in hospital settings, a preoccupation with hospitals is not unfounded in a discussion of staff nurse collegiality. Within a hospital, each patient care unit is a structure within the organization, just as each hospital is a part of the Ontario Hospitals Association (OHA). The type of contact between hospitals is one of competition, with linkages through the OHA. As we will discuss later in this chapter, however, it is the way in which the OHA, which bargains with the nurses' union, the Ontario Nurses Association (ONA) that impacts on the staff nurse's role. During the period of this research, and even today, hospitals reduced and re-engineered their employees, put in place new work procedures, and restructured their institutions, all of which contributed to workload increases for nurses at the bedside. As most of my survey research was conducted in the first years of hospital "downsizing" in 1994, issues related to current hospital restructuring were not at issue. Therefore, although health care restructuring issues are referred to within this chapter, these were not a major part of the research, and will not be addressed at length. The focus is primarily on the structures that affect the staff nurse's work environment, the nursing image (Muff 1982), and the relationships that occur within this environment.

Organizational structure is a framework for working relationships among members of a system, and for the nursing profession this includes, not only the government which funds health care, but also the CNO, RNAO, OHA, and ONA. The manner in which each part acts and interacts with the other provides values and norms, and establishes organizational communications. Due to outcome strategies that are part of governance models adopted by the OHA and individual hospitals, these organizations also have input into, and make decisions that affect the RN working at the bedside.

The concept of structure is about decision-making as characterized by Bess (1988), and staff nurses are not represented at this level. The inter-actions that occur among these organizations are established in keeping with the goals of each organization, and the staff nurse is not a major player but depends on those in management positions to represent the interest of nursing. Although there are differences in mandate that separate the four member organizations that comprise the structure of nursing, the relations between them can be viewed as a single macro structure which makes possible the identification of the decision-making power and patterns each component of this structure has and uses to the benefit or disadvantage of the staff nurse.

Thus, when viewed structurally, the profession of nursing is comprised of a number of relational organizations, which includes profes-sional education/training (colleges and universities), professional associa-tions (RNAO), professional colleges (CNO), and professional bargaining units/unions (ONA). Together, they form the architecture of the macro structure, wherein nurses communicate at an organizational level with each other, and are engaged in managing the system. If we were to only consider organizations involved directly in nursing, the OHA would not be included. While the OHA represents hospitals, it does influence what occurs within the profession of nursing in Ontario. This is the case in part because hospi-tals traditionally were the institutions that trained and socialized nurses when the occupation was first developed (Bingham 1979). Although no longer assigned the task of educating and training nurses in Ontario, hospi-tals have maintained a voice in nursing practice when it comes to nurses working in acute care, as they are the major employer of Registered Nurses.[1] Universities and colleges do, however, provide the initial socializa-tion of nurses, and academic leaders from universities and colleges have input, first through the RNAO, as members of that organization, and secondly, as experts providing advice to the CNO and the Ministry of Health (MOH). In this manner, as well as through their writings, nurses in educational roles influence the role of the staff nurse. Nursing organizations are also involved in advocating nursing excellence, and professional stan-dards, even though they each play a different role, and provide different viewpoints when interacting within the structure and with the MoH. This chapter will discuss the four organizations named above.

In the literature of organizational theory, structure is typically defined as a pattern or design by which institutions are organized and integrated, as well as activities and communications conducted through the structure itself (Bess 1988, 97). Considering the variety of functions and interests that occur within the profession of nursing, the structure of decision making—of how and who makes decisions—will influence the culture within which nurses work, and by association the culture of collegiality. The competing viewpoints of the four organizations that occupy positions within the profession of nursing can promote or block change that affects the staff nurse working within the hospital.

The hospital is also a player through its senior nursing administrators as they have input into the professional structure through the RNAO. Hospitals then play a major part in the system of professional nursing, first, through their nursing managerial staff who usually belong to the RNAO, as well as through the OHA in dealing with issues concerning nurses. The MoH, through its policies, lends power to the OHA in its relationship to nurses' work. These separate groups are co-ordinated through formal interaction, as well as through informal networking. The arrangement and participation of these formal groups, as well as structures external to the environment of nursing, such as the MoH, provide the material conditions for working, for beliefs, and for values that produce or hinder the culture of collegiality within the nursing profession.

Nursing has a distinct subculture, one traditionally symbolized in the past by a white uniform, cap, and pin.[2] Contemporary socialization processes, their educational philosophies, and concomitant ideological underpinnings provide nurses with a distinct subculture of caring that is inherited from the past (Boykin 1995). Stakeholders within nursing have largely replaced such symbols with notions of professionalism and collegiality, concepts in which caring is viewed as important. The communication of this conceptual identity among nurses occurs through the agency of organization like the RNAO, the CNO, and the ONA. Through the ONA, staff nurses have a formal organization that can address their concerns when the other stakeholders connect professionalism to higher entry-level university trained nurses and when government and hospitals discuss their economic worth. Hospitals and governments play a role when discussing the worth of nurses in economic terms when it comes to collective bargaining. The staff nurses are not part of the macro structure and we must attend to their absence from this structure in any discussion of their true role in the

---

health care system. We know that without the staff nurse, hospitals could not function. Seen as essential workers, government has taken away their right to strike from the collective bargaining process. The RNAO and ONA speak to this issue of "worth," but their voices have limited success because these two organizations act individually and in their own self-interest.

Gender difference in this structure is of some relevance. The RNAO, the ONA, and the CNO are governed by women who were socialized within the profession of nursing, while the OHA and most hospitals have male administrators usually holding MBA degrees and are socialized outside of the nursing profession. As most administrators and medical chiefs of hospitals are male, and as nursing administrators are female, the gendered power distribution of society at large is replicated within the structure of relations of nursing that is under examination here. In addition, within nursing management, white women occupy most positions, even though there are competent racialised nurses working at the staff nurse level and an increase in the number of visible minority patients. White nurse leaders speak about male dominance and patriarchy while remaining blind to their racist behaviours and the white privilege they enjoy.

The three nursing organizations in this structure are discussed here in terms of their attention to political strategies and how these strategies relate to the Ministry of Health. The MoH is the main source of power in the health care system. The manner in which these organizations relate to this source provides the organizations in turn with power, which translates into how decisions are made within the structure of nursing. The ethno-cultural differences between the rulers and the ruled within the nursing profession provide for some of the distance between the two groupings. Most nursing leaders within the profession come from the dominant ethnic group in the wider society, while those at the bedside are from racialised groups or are new immigrants (Hagey et al. 2005).

Formal identity for nurses as a group is maintained or changed through the major institutions involved in the profession. The four organizations form the structure wherein decisions are made as to what nursing means and what it undertakes as a profession within the province of Ontario. The outcomes of their relationships influence the work behaviour of the staff nurse group and their shared identity, which also arises from the nature of the work nurses do when employed in a hospital. The concept of collegiality and, by association, the understanding of "nursing structure," is central to understanding "the culture of nursing collegiality." The way the profession is structured influences the professional culture, and produces collegial and/or conflictual behaviour.

Through the lens of power and authority (Weber 1946), each 'player' within the system and the dynamics that occur between these four groups can be analysed. The span of control and power that each part has within the structure produces coalitions that shift and move according to the positions each organization has on a particular issue. Power in this chapter is viewed then as how each part of the system affects the other's behaviour, and influences their situation or position. This is so, both within the overall structure, and also in the health care system in general. This positioning in the healthcare system is conceived as a more pervasive and important way of exercising power (Ritzer 1990) than is unwilling compliance or force. The four organizations in the profession of nursing have levels of legitimate authority defined by laws and regulations that account for the roles they play within the structure of the profession, and the interactions that they have with individual staff nurses.

External forces such as public opinion, funding, government attitudes around health care, and nurses all influence the stakeholders within the system. This affects the structure of the nursing profession, and in turn affects staff nurses. By recognizing the power of government to approve and implement broad health care policies, we can focus on the 'players' whose mission and activities exert influence on the profession in their day-to-day activities. An understanding of the organizations which strongly influences the culture of nursing in Ontario will contextualize the behaviour detected at the staff nurse level, which is also based on social roles learned while in university or college, or both.

The Four Organizations:
Their Visions and Interactions Within the Profession

In the life of a staff nurses, the two major organizations that have power over their day-to-day activities are the CNO and—through the institution in which she or he works—the OHA. Supporting them within the profession, and adding their voices, is the RNAO and the ONA. The MoH provides healthcare funding and establishes the overall policy framework, which influences all of the organizations under discussion here, thereby influencing the work-life of the staff nurse.

The College of Nurses of Ontario (CNO)

The mandate of the CNO states that it exists to protect the public interest. The involvement of the Canadian Nursing Association (CNA) through the Board of Directors (Kerr and MacPhail 1996) has resulted in the development of standards for nursing care in Canada that influence CNO policies. This association has also provided input into the development of mandatory registration and into the overall scope of nursing practice, which then influences the CNO. The College receives its authority under the Regulated Health Professions Act (1994), the Nursing Act (1991), and the Procedural Code. Created in 1962, the College was given the responsibility by government of supervising schools of nursing, registration, and disciplinary functions, which had been previously handled by the RNAO's Board of Directors. This governing body for registered nurses provides the graduate nurse with a valid Certification of Registration, in order that he or she may work within the province of Ontario. The CNO's professional standards can be understood as legitimating claims to self-regulation and professionalism. This symbolism of self-regulation hooks in with the bureaucratic organization of work.

The CNO, as a bureaucratic organization, places many constraints on its members that hinder their active participation in the development of regulatory policy. In 1994, under the Regulated Health Professions Act (RHPA), the CNO became responsible for developing and maintaining programmes and standards of practice to assure the quality of practice of the profession. A majority of nurses in Ontario have a vague image of the College of Nurses as an entity, located in Toronto, that makes "the rules" and disciplines members who err (*Communiquè*, May 1998). In principle, the RHPA gives autonomy to the CNO and gives nurses the right to practice their profession. This provides for role autonomy, and nurses must define what they can do, and what they cannot do, in relation to the stipulations of the Act. Most members keep an arms-length approach to the CNO, and view it as the body that sets requirements for entrance to the profession, establishes and enforces standards of nursing practice, and assures the quality of practice of the profession, and the continuing competence of nurses.

Although the College validates nurses as professionals, it is the enforcement aspect of the CNO that makes many staff nurses reluctant to participate within the CNO in the various projects that the organization undertakes. Although the CNO states that the standards empower the nurse to be free to make her or his own decisions, it is particularly around this point that conflict between the environment of professionalism and the bureaucratic model within which nurses' work occurs. The professional model accords the RN autonomy and responsibility to make decisions through standards of patient care. While the bureaucratic model is an efficient means of handling large numbers of individuals in giving service within actions that are rationally organized within an institution. Thus, there is a clash between these two cultures—the culture of professionalism, and the bureaucratic organization in which the nurse is employed. Nevertheless, nurses find themselves drawing upon the values and norms of the professional culture within the hospital.[3]

The CNO has not played a major role in addressing issues resulting from health sector "downsizing," nor does it provide the OHA with an ideal nurse-to-patient ratio. It also does not provide specifications of what constitutes an unsafe condition for registered nurses to practice nursing within an institution, even though nurses can report unsafe institutional conditions to the CNO. When the CNO investigates written complaints about the nursing practice and conduct of its members, the allegations can be reviewed in conjunction with the nurse's report to the CNO on the same issue. The CNO has power over its members but lacks the power to direct the MoH and the OHA on issues important to patient care involving nurses. When cutbacks have occurred that have impacted on the nursing profession and patient care, it has not used public opinion to embarrass these organizations.

The College of Nursing of Ontario is one of the major agents of socialization for nurses throughout their careers. Staff nurses are aware of standards through the CNO and their education system. Through their Quality Assurance Program, the CNO encourages nursing professionals to update knowledge and skills, and to maintain competence throughout their nursing careers. Thus, the College sets the standards for professionalism and professional behaviour. As such, it places nurses in the position to police one another's performance. Such surveillance of, and reporting on a colleague, runs counter, however, to collegial behaviour. Although other professions have policies regarding the reporting of colleagues, nursing has a reporting culture based on the reporting of medication errors. Nurses must fill in forms regarding any mistakes they find, and submit these forms to their managers, who at their discretion may report them to the CNO.

The CNO also contributes to the socialization of nurses by providing a monthly publication in respect to how nurses need to conduct themselves towards the public. The codifying of collective identities is accomplished by publishing documents designed to explain nursing relationships and in examining the actions of the nurse. For example, the College's *Communiqué* publishes verbatim the Discipline Committee of the CNO's decisions, and their rationale. They state:

> Identifying information revealing the names of witnesses and patients and location of the incident(s) has been removed. It is hoped that by publishing these decisions in full it will educate the public as to what is deemed inappropriate nursing practice. Of added benefit to the public is that these decisions will also educate RNs and RPNs as to what is appropriate behaviour when they find themselves in similar situations. (*Communiqué*, October 1993, 26)

The name of the staff nurse and the penalty for the professional misconduct that occurred is published in the *Communiqué*, although the Registered Nurse has the right to make an appeal to the Divisional Court of Ontario. Under the RHPA, any citizen in Ontario can obtain the results of every disciplinary and incapacity proceeding that has been completed. If an individual calls the College seeking information on a particular member, the College will provide whatever information is available on the public register. Some members feel that their safety could be at risk, and that the business address should not become public without some safeguards. This rationale is based on the possibility that someone, such as a former patient or an ex-spouse, could, through the College, track down a nurse who, for the reasons of safety, may not wish to be located. Understanding this as a safety issue, the College will seek permission of the specific member prior to revealing information of the individual's whereabouts. In organizations where professionals are the main focus, the problems of accommodating bureaucratic control and professionalism present difficulties to the members, on account of the authority relationship that exists. Thus, the role of the CNO puts it in a position of power and authority over nurses, yet it lacks power to stand up for them when they work in unsafe situations.

The CNO has traditionally influenced the workplace by promoting and maintaining standards of practice, but it does not have the power to investigate hospitals in terms of nursing care to patient ratios, nor does it have jurisdiction over the hiring practices, the monitoring of human rights standards, or staffing patterns of individual hospitals. Nurses who are managers and administrators can be investigated if involved in an unsafe work environment incidents occurs, and if patient safety is threatened. Most of the complaints are, however, staff nurse related.

Although acknowledging a distinction between employment-related concerns and those related to substandard practice, unprofessional conduct, or incapacity due to illness, the CNO in actuality does little about employment-related concerns. It becomes involved only if a report or a complaint were to be lodged against a nurse administrator. In my years of acute care practice, I have seen that the policies and procedures that hospitals have in place have provided a shield for senior nursing administrators against investigation by the College. Managers in nursing can simply cite a policy in order to avoid investigation. Conversely, policies allow for judgements to be made about a staff nurse who can be questioned as to why she or he did not follow a particular policy, or make allowance for extenuating circumstances.

The CNO derives its authority from the Health Disciplines Act, the mandate of which is to serve and protect the public interest. According to that Act, any employer of a RN is legally obligated to report to the College any termination that has occurred for reasons that might constitute professional misconduct. The rationale underlying this reporting process is that the public interest is potentially safeguarded. The link between the hospital and the College is a reporting one and is governed by law; thus, the CNO's power and authority derive from what Weber called "legal authority" (Weber 1946, 328). Prior to enacting or revising standards through the *Communiqué*, comments and critiques are gathered from the membership. This mode of consultation has a legitimizing effect on governance, however, the feeling among staff nurses is that the College is a punitive body, and thus nurses have not built any type of partnership with the organization as individuals. In fact, when white managers target them, racialised nurses, view the allegations brought before the College as backlash (Hagey et al. 2005). They feel that these managers do not report their white peers for the same behaviours, and thus believe that they are being targeted. This lack of trust and the governance of the College by mostly white persons bring forward the question of legitimacy in how decisions are made. On behalf of its membership, the ONA has an interactive relationship with the

CNO, and represents members when allegations occur. The CNO views itself as successful in building partnerships with healthcare organizations, nursing employers, nursing educators, the government, and the consumers, in order to influence the competing interests at play (*Communiqué*, December 1997, 6).

The voices in the *Communiqué* are those from the dominant group, and it is these women who, within organizations, hold managerial power, or are educators, and researchers. When enacting or revising standards, it is the powerful stakeholders that get heard, as they participate directly in committees and discussion groups, and not the staff nurses working at the bedside who tend not to participate. Although difficult to prove conclusively, from the point of view of staff nurses and of a participant observer, decisions are not made in a democratic way; pre-regulatory "consultation" is viewed as an ideological, legitimating exercise on the part of agents of the macro structure.

With effective collaboration, the CNO can only strengthen its own role in the workplace with the staff nurse group, as they currently view the College as ineffective when it comes to their work environment. The College does not have legal authority to set standards for patient-staff ratios in hospitals, or to sanction hospitals when they harass, or do not act in the best interest of their staff. This was evident for example, during the SARS outbreak, and it further irritates staff nurses who feel that they put their lives on the line just by going to work. The CNO is clearly not seen as a body that protects the nurse from the employer but rather, as an entity that protects patients from nurses.

The structure of the profession is managed through a formal system of authority that is not collegial in the common sense of the term (Bess 1988, 99); bureaucratic authority runs counter to collegiality, as the latter involves integrated, participatory decision-making. In Bess's view, superiors can expedite decisions based on their particular expertise. Given standardization of professional preparation, CNO accountability, and legal, rational authority, standards and disciplines provide for the culture of collegiality.

The Ontario Hospital Association (OHA)

Although a voluntary association, the OHA represents more than two hundred public hospitals. Administrators from these hospitals are the main players within this association; they are major players in the nursing professional structure, as the OHA's decisions impacts on nurses working within the hospital. The OHA is influential in developing and promoting a united front for hospitals when they need to speak to the government on what it recognizes as improvements for patient care within the industry. Since all hospitals and long-term care facilities are members of this organization, they speak with one voice, and over the years, have been empowered by the media. This association also received legal, rational power from the Joint Policy and Planning Committee (JPPC), which was established in 1992.

The JPPC was formed as a partnership between the Ministry of Health (MoH) and the OHA, and is co-chaired by the Deputy Minister of Health and the Board Chair of the OHA. It has a mandate to recommend and aid the implementation of hospital reform. The direct link that the OHA has to the Ministry provides this organization, which represents hospitals, with power to affect the direction of policy in health care. At the time of writing, with changes in the health care system, the provincial government is attempting to legislate a new structure through Bill 36, the Local Health Integration Networks (LHINs), in order to promote accountability and integration based upon resource allocation. If passed, hospitals will have to interact with this community network for strategic direction.

Through the OHA's Public Affairs and Educational Division, the OHA provides continuing education, and a strategic and co-ordinated focus on communications and government relations. It also has formal links to professional organizations, including nursing. This liaison is for the benefit of issues of management, education, and policy development (OHA 1997). The OHA plays a major role within the nursing profession as the spokesperson and negotiator for the employer. Senior nursing administrators have influence in directing the profession through the RNAO as well as the OHA. This type of linkage is comparable to corporate interlocking directorships. For example, a past president of the RNAO was a senior administrator in a large teaching hospital in Toronto. This individual had access to the OHA as a part of hospital administration, had links to the MoH when dealing with health policy, and the CNO because of her position, both at the RNAO, and in her role as a hospital administrator. As part of hospital administration, she brings to the RNAO the administrative views of nursing and the interest of the OHA.

The work lives of staff nurses are affected by the outcomes of the policy decisions that the OHA makes. The OHA has direct input and participation in the JPPC, and speaks for the hospital administration, enabling this administration to shape and influence policy for nursing within the health care system by co-operating with the Ministry at all levels. The JPPC *Profile* (1998) shows effective relationships with several key stakeholders, which includes the College of Physicians and Surgeons of Ontario, and the Ontario Medical Association (OMA). It does not include the CNO or ONA, which means that nurses are not directly represented by their associations or college. This type of governing process is replicated within hospitals where the Chief of Medical Staff is included on the Board, while the Chief of Nursing is not a voting member. Hospitals receive their budgets from the MoH, and can use tax dollars to promote their concerns. Thus, in terms of economic power, the hospitals have far more economic power than the three other organizations in the JPPC, which rely solely on membership dues.

Like ONA, the OMA is a union for the medical profession within the Ontario health system, yet it is included in the working relationships with the JPPC. By being included, both the OHA and the MoH have contributed to the marginalization of nurses within the health system. The OHA is empowered through its membership, and creates new power for its members through the JPPC. It can be argued that nurses are represented through nursing divisions within hospitals. Senior nurses within hospitals are, however, part of the administrative team, and when making decisions around nursing care within hospitals, speak for the administration, not for the profession.

A good example of this can be seen in the fact that ONA's views on such issues as funding approaches are different from those of the JPPC; the JPPC's viewpoint includes those of hospital and senior nurse administrators. Discussions are centred around financial concerns of the hospital sector, as was demonstrated by the "downsizing" of health care workers by hospitals. The MoH is influenced by this lobbying far more than the concerns of ONA around what is to be done in relation to this workforce and about how the workforce should be structured. ONA's evolving vision is built upon the five pillars of the Canada Health Act (ONA 1996) and which is also the mandate of the provincial government.

The authority that hospitals have in hiring and firing nurses creates a relationship of command and obedience. Nurses have become the primary target for the achievement of cost savings in the health care system. Moreover, nurses state that the OHA blames them, as does the Minister for having asked for and successfully negotiated a decent wage increase of 2%

(ONA n.d.). For example, those in senior management positions within the hospitals had received salary increases between 13 to 46%. At that time, the Ontario government wanted wages to stay flat, or to increase at a rate of 2%. The actions of the hospitals in the area of salary increases for upper management created conflict with the government's position for workers, yet the government did not take action, or make comments when hospitals increased salaries for senior management.

Hospitals convey to the community the importance of their role in the health care system. Empowered by the public perception of their role, hospitals have lacked accountability when dealing with staff nurses, and have, with impunity, replaced them with non-professional workers, such as health care aids. The public has accepted the various non-professional care-givers that now work within the hospital system.

The shortage of nurses and the lack of continuity of care are all blamed on the lack of funding rather than looking at how funds that are received from the MoH are allocated. When questioned in the Collegiality Survey about the importance of their role within the hospital, 12.4% of nurses surveyed stated that hospital management always viewed their role as important in the functioning of the hospital. When taking the "often" (31%) and "sometimes" (38.8%) categories together, 69.8% of staff nurses feel that hospital management has viewed them as important some of the time. When discussing the actions of hospitals in hiring and firing staff nurses and replacing them with health care aids, nurses stated that the lack of respect for their role is evident in the decisions made by administration. They point to the situation of budget controls, and when the staff-patient ratio is not discussed with them.

In general, I found that staff nurses resented the professional struc-ture, and associated those in administration with the structure. They also associated their lack of power with the MoH's dealings with the administra-tion and the fact that they did not take the staff nurses' views into account. Those at the administrative level speak to patient care issues without under-standing the day-to-day activities that are performed by their employees, and made decisions that are not in the interest of patient care but are moti-vated by a corporate agenda. Moreover, nurses believe that their contribu-tion to the hospital is devalued by the administration. It is instructive that 17.5% of the nurses in the sample stated that they thought that the admin-istration always took care of itself at the expense of the staff nurse. When this percentage is added to those numbers that fall within the "often" and "sometimes" categories, the result is a total of 87.4% who hold a view of hospital administration as taking care of its own needs at the expense of the employee.

Staff nurses saw in their daily reality, the increased power and salaries of hospital administrators that has been gained over the years while their own workload increased without proper remuneration. The following statement represents the attitude of many staff nurses:

> We are working harder; the managers are nowhere to be found, always in meetings or in their office. They spend money on what they see as important. They cut back on the RPNs [Registered Practical Nurses] and want all RNs, and then they cut the RNs and bring in the Aids who help do the heavy tasks. But now they will bring back the RPNs. All this cost money that they pay out in packages. I am finding that I have to check that the work gets done because with the bumping that takes place we get new staff who do not know the unit. As soon as we get settled, the musical chairs start again, and the unit is always in chaos. We also have less staff. I think someone in a university thinks about these changes, writes a paper, and then these ideas are picked up by those in nursing management. (O.S., surgical staff nurse)

While staff nurses, like the one quoted above, tie changes that take place to research at the university level, the nursing administration usually ties the changes that they implement to the lack of funding from the government.

The change in models of care are implemented without input from staff nurses but are designed by Nurse Managers. Management nurses are not the ones that provide care but get the go ahead from senior administrators to change from team nursing to primary nursing, or to another model. Year after year, models of care have changed, and lay-off packages have been traditionally provided. Staff nurses view the process of buying out nurses when terminating them and then rehiring them when the model is changed as a waste of resources. They witness new staff hired for a different category level of nursing to take the place of those "de-hired," "let go," "or given a package."

The process usually follows the following cycle: from team nursing to primary nursing, and then back to a type of team nursing. The

Collegiality Survey shows that when changes occur, staff nurses think that their views are not canvassed before changes take place. Only 2.3% of staff nurses thought that administration always ask for their views before implementing changes that affect them, while 19.2% think that they never get asked for their input. Nurses have come to see their labour as expendable and see those in management maintaining an edge on power over the staff nurses.

During restructuring, hospitals held consultation forums for their staff. Nurses expressed their views in these forums; however, they and other employees distrusted all of the major players in the structure, and felt the same level of distrust in the government. Announcements from the government add to this distrust and distress. In March 1999, the Government of Ontario announced the need for 12,000 nursing jobs in Ontario. In 2004 the Government of Ontario announced that 700 nursing jobs in Ontario were to be eliminated. In terms of nursing care, the Government makes decisions without the participation of the staff nurse group (including ONA). Such lack of consultation promotes distrust towards government and also leaves staff nurses feeling vulnerable in their daily work-lives.

The lack of input from nurses at the hospital level, and the fact that the ONA does not have standing at the JPPC, places the ONA at a disadvantage when changes are made that affect nurses. Staff nurses are aware that the OHA represents hospitals, and that the OHA battles with the ONA in collective bargaining—the OHA represents the hospital within the system while the ONA represents the nurse within the system. The very nature of the relationship between the employer and the union is one of conflict, each viewing the transformation of the system with different agendas.

The decisions that the ONA makes in relation to the OHA around staffing issues and grievances are hospital specific. When a hospital fails to provide a safe work environment, and refuses to look into work-related issues, the ONA censures these institutions. It then publishes the name of the censured hospital, and informs the College of what has taken place. When the hospital rectifies the problems and tries to ensure a safe working environment, the hospital is taken off the list.

In my interviews around this issue, I was informed that most hospitals that the ONA is involved with do not want to be censured. For example, one hospital in Toronto that had been censured in early 1990, worked on their relationship with their nurses, and with the ONA. In so doing, the ONA was able to de-list the hospital, and commented that they had become

71

a stellar organization to deal with, in terms of employee relationships. The power to shame provides the ONA with the ability to expose how hospitals set patient-staff ratios, and how nursing grievances are handled, especially when they do not abide by their own policies. Nurses report these discrepancies to ONA, and this gives ONA the power to investigate work-related injuries, and also when the hospital refuses to provide alternative work for injured employees. Through the censuring mechanism, ONA has the ability to take the employer to various tribunals (such as the WSIB) and to more generally monitor the labour relations within the hospital work environment.

The ONA, the CNO, and the MoH have little formal input into budgetary allocation for registered nurses within a hospital. The OHA also does not have policy guidelines or policies for hospitals in terms of a patient-staff ratio, nor in terms of which type of caregiver provides care to patients in the hospital. Administrators and hospital boards within each hospital spend tax dollars on issues that they deem important, usually according to a strategic plan and without true consultation with their community.

There have been attempts within hospitals to find out through quality assurance programmes, and data collection, whether or not patients are receiving adequate care. When reviewing how resources are divided in a health care facility, administrators look at how to cut back on highly paid registered nurses, and how to replace them with lower-paid staff. While discussing the issue of administrative action with a staff nurse, she informed me that a majority of nurses like her do not feel included in the decisions that affect them within the hospital where they work. She said:

> They give a great party and package for presidents who
> leave, while those who work their backsides off do not get
> the same acknowledgment for their work when they leave.
> (O.S., staff nurse, medical)

The Harris Government in Ontario provided the names and salaries of those individuals within the hospital sector who earn more than $100,000. Called the "Sunshine law," these figures are published annually in newspapers. Although this made the public aware of administrators' incomes, there is neither public outrage nor a backlash; and as it is a one-day issue in the media, this information is soon forgotten. The negative optics of management going to conventions and increasing their salaries provides for a view of an administrative body that is insular, and unaccountable.

In this survey, respondents believed that even when hospital administrators saw their role as important, these same administrators took care of their own needs at the expense of the staff. While discussing her work environment, a staff nurse said:

> Who asked the bedside nurse for their input into policy while nurse educators and nurse management review articles and data to make policy that affects their staff who do the work? All these meetings... you go to meetings where administration asks for our ideas but they do what they want anyway. (V.D., staff nurse, psychiatry, January 1996)

This alienation from decision making and a view of a "greedy" administration provides a work environment in which staff nurses do not see themselves or their union as participating in the process of resource allocation. To nurses, this spells out the difference between the two levels of thinking that are distinct from each other within the hospital environment.

Media coverage has portrayed the hospital sector as an industry that is hard-done by, through lack of funding by government. Little effort is given by the media to acquaint their readers with cost-saving abilities in home-care, how hospitals are managed, and the wait time for cardiac care, and cancer care. The media gets its information by relying solely on the messages that the OHA, the MoH, and other agencies provide them. Through its public relations office, the OHA speaks to the media about the lack of government funding and about how programmes have to be downsized. CBC News (September 7, 2004) reported that "...they check your blood pressure, they give you pills, they clean you and they comfort you. They're nurses - and in Canada, they're tired, worn out, and fed up." At times, when dealing with nursing care, the media does not try to differentiate between those who work at the bedside and those nurses who teach and manage patient care. They seem unaware that hospitals have more layers within nursing care after restructuring, and did not cut back on managers.

Cut-backs in service takes place at the bedside, and as their numbers diminish, staff nurses see the hiring of Case Managers, Nurse Educators, Risk Managers, Clinical Nurse Specialists and Nurse Clinicians, even when hospitals state that they lack funds. Hospital Managers will cut programs, blaming the lack of funding while simultaneously hiring people into these nursing positions. Once again, this misunderstanding of how funds are spent shows the hospital's power through the OHA in getting out its message, and the lack of collaboration among the ONA and the RNAO to provide an alternate message around the role of the staff nurse.

The MoH is currently also trying to communicate to the public regarding the availability of community care, and the new regional funding; the message is drowned out, however, by stories in the media of patients in emergency departments not receiving care, and how the system is falling apart. The public still perceives hospitals as the main focus in the delivery of services within the health care system, and listens to the media's message of what is needed within that system.

The RNAO

When the CNO was created in 1962, the RNAO, founded as a voluntary professional organization, representing both supervisory and staff nurses, lost the power to regulate education, to register, to examine, and to discipline nurses within Ontario. The RNAO has a long history of encouraging public policies that support and promote health, and views itself as the professional association that fosters the role of nursing within the health care system in Ontario. As an independent, voluntary association, the RNAO tries to provide a voice for registered nurses through active involvement in policy analysis, education, professional development, and a legal assistance program for its members. Involvement in the RNAO offers opportunities to join interest groups such as Mental Health, Nurse Administrators, and Critical Care, and to participate in sub-committees and workshops. The RNAO has 20,475 members (RNAO 2004) out of the 105,739 Registered Nurses in Ontario (CNO 2004).

Higher levels of nursing management still have influence in this organization, which refused to act as the central bargaining unit for nurses because it did not want to shut off higher levels of managerial nurses from its own membership (Armstrong, Choiniere, and Day 1993, 99). The president of RNAO is a member who has links to hospital administrators and to university colleagues, and is usually from the dominant group in society. The Provincial Nursing Administrators Interest Group, an interest group of the RNAO, has members who are presidents of hospitals, or professors in universities. The ties between the RNAO and upper management in hospitals derive from this interest group, and from members of the Board.

During restructuring, the RNAO viewed budget cuts and hospital closings as a threat to access to services, but did not censure or shame senior nursing administrators when they developed inferior care models. They stated in part:

A bottom-line mentality has promoted an indiscriminate replacement of registered nurses by less-prepared health care providers. As a result, registered nurses are experiencing a dramatic decrease in the time available for direct patient care. (RNAO n.d., 1)

In the 1990s, as a public awareness tactic, both the public and registered nurses were encouraged to document their personal stories, and to send them to the RNAO. This was one way of gathering information, which could be used on the internet or in other public forums. Letters to the media regarding generic workers as a quick-fix that would not save hospitals money and would be detrimental to patents, fact sheets about hospital restructuring, meetings with MPPs, and other political action were all part of an ongoing process to influence and promote "healthy public policy" (November 1997). The RNAO perceives itself as a strong, credible voice for the nursing profession but does not use its voice to influence nursing leaders to rethink working conditions for the RN within their institutions. The professionalism of nursing can be viewed as a focal point in its message to the public, and to the MoH.

The RNAO views nursing as a knowledge profession, wherein the nurse makes critical decisions regarding patient care, and handles exacting procedures and medications within increasingly complex social settings. This organization is very supportive of the move by the CNO to identify a new set of competency expectations for new registered nurses. It announced: "Beginning in January 2005, a baccalaureate degree in nursing will be the minimum education expectation for Ontario applicants who are entering the profession" (RNAO 1999, 8). Clearly, for the RNAO, educational reform is in the best interest of the public, for nursing in general, and for nurses (RNAO 1999, 14).

Although this organization acknowledges the shortage of registered nurses, and the reduction of students entering the profession, it does not view its stand on educational reform as a deterrent to women entering the work force at the college level. In reviewing the goal of a baccalaureate degree in nursing, the RNAO does not address what would happen to new immigrant women holding diploma certificates rather than university degrees.

In Healthy Work Environments Best Practice Guidelines Project (RNAO website 2005) the RNAO states that it wants to maximize the health and well-being of nurses, quality patient outcomes, and organizational performance, without commenting on dysfunctional nurse-nurse relationships. The organisation has also not addressed the overall lack of minorities in leadership positions in both nursing administration and education, as well as the lack of role models for ethnic minority nursing students (see Purzan 2003).

Although the RNAO may speak out at times against abuse, harassment, and racism, it appears to be unaware of how policies can affect those who are not members of the dominant group. In a rush towards professionalism, the elites within the profession may leave their minority sisters behind. Perhaps they are also unaware that this may cause new immigrant RNs to become under-employed as Health Care Aids, or reduced to positions of as RPNs (Registered Practical Nurses) due to the lack of a university degree.

The Ontario Nurses Association (ONA)

Due to the refusal of the RNAO to become the bargaining unit for staff nurses, the ONA was formed in 1973. Misinformation spread by the hospital and the RNAO regarding the role of ONA as compared to that of the RNAO confused staff nurses when they voted to become unionized. Hospitals promoted membership in the RNAO by adding such membership to a list of requirements when advertising positions. The ONA currently represents fifty thousand members across the province of Ontario; they work in hospitals, nursing homes, homes for the aged, public health, community clinics, home care programmes, and the Victorian Order of Nurses (VON) (ONA 1993).

The ONA is a trade union that bargains collectively for improved working conditions and wages and is also active in the promotion of the profession itself. The Ontario Labour Relations Act (LRA) determines which nurses are included in and excluded from this bargaining unit. The ONA assists members in matters of contract interpretations, contract enforcement, and patient care concerns, and focuses more on the working environment for nurses within the hospital system. The union provides several insurance policies for its members, including malpractice insurance. It represents its members before government Task Forces and Commissions, lobbies the government for health care reform, and provides submissions to the CNO, suggesting improvements to the Standards of Practice.

Staff nurses are not engaged in their union and the voting turnout is low. They view the union as needed but are unable to deal with the racism and abuse within it, that they consider to be aimed at them. Racialised nurses view union leaders as mostly white, and not in touch with their issues.

To solve the funding crisis in health care, the OHA with approval from the government (1996a, 1), has asked nurses to take a greater than twenty per cent cut in their wages. According to the ONA (1996a), nurses have become the primary target to achieve cost savings in the health care system. Using this issue and the cutbacks that have occurred, the ONA has been educating its membership about the current realities. They reveal that their membership feel neglected, ignored, and taken advantage of by their employers (1996a, 2). This is understandable, given that the hospital system has eliminated five thousand nursing positions, and has shifted many nurses from full-time status to part-time positions.

Even as recently as 2005, the provincial government has targeted registered nurses' positions as a means of saving on health care expenses. With these cuts added to the past elimination of nursing positions, we find a demoralized group of staff nurses who feel rushed, and are unable to provide the nursing care that their patients should receive. Political activity is not a part of most staff nurses' agenda: tired and overworked, they do their jobs and go home.

As part of ONA's 1996 Annual Meeting activities, more than one thousand delegates joined up with consumers, nurse colleagues, and health-care allies in a march on the provincial legislature at Queen's Park, (ONA, Queen's Park March). The march was organized as political action by the union, and to give staff nurses a public voice. Using its Annual Meeting as a linkage, ONA invited Duncan Sinclair, Chair of the Provincial Health Services Restructuring Commission, to be its keynote speaker. The following excerpt from his speech is useful for the purposes of this discussion:

> ONA has shown itself to be doing its part to shape the future
> for health care. They have sought to meet with us and bring

forward a proposal for health reform that will mean a system that is more accessible, high quality and more affordable, in the context of the real world, for many, many years. ONA has communicated its solution far and wide. What I say to ONA is—keep it up. (ONA's 23 Annual Meeting)

In order to represent its membership, the ONA has developed a process to determine their views as accurately as possible before bargaining begins. By 1980, ninety-two percent of hospitals were participating in the central bargaining process. It is in this environment that staff nurses have the opportunity to work together within a collegial framework because the ONA demonstrated that the staff nurses' interest is its main priority. As an organization, the ONA has a role to represent its members in areas such as heath restructuring. In helping to create a vision of a high quality health care system, the ONA recognized, as did Dr. Sinclair, that it is an organization speaking for nurses.

The ONA's power comes not only from the Ontario Labour Relations Act but also from its large membership who understand that "if nurses want to change this system, they are going to have to mobilize" (ONA 1996a, 1). Understanding the power of communication, the ONA launched a campaign that involved thousands of nurses in dialogue with their colleagues in health care, and with the public. "Nurses are going to tell the truth about what's going on," said ONA's CEO. "And when they do, they'll let the government and those responsible at the community level know what they think" (1996a, 3).

As a membership-driven organization, the ONA was, and is recognized as a leader within the health care system, both because it seeks public-interest solutions that are evidenced-based, and because it advocates for model workplaces that are free from harassment and discrimination. It fosters understanding and trust among ONA, the RNAO, and the College of Nurses through liaising and through continuing collaboration with other nurses' unions across Canada. It has also gone on record as sharing in the collection of research and data (ONA Statement of Beliefs 2005) (ONA, Organizational Transformation 1997, 2). If the voices of nurses are to be heard, it will have to happen through the collective action of many individual nurses through their organization.

At the Unit Level

Staff nurses' work is visible, and provides an opportunity for the observer to formulate judgements about the work that nurses do. At the unit level, staff nurses have an environment that is based on expectations such as: "patients first," answering call bells quickly, emptying bedpans, being a handmaiden to the physician, "Tender Loving Care" (TLC) providers, and medication dispensers. The image of the nurse is entrenched in the minds of the public — the patients and families that come to hospitals for treatment, as well as those who work within the hospital. Thus, what goes on at the unit level is at times removed from the organizational structure itself and is more focused on immediate patient needs. On the other hand, the determining of the nurse's role can be attributed to all of these sources: administrative channels, such as the CNO, the OHA; the expectations of immediate colleagues; subordinates, and peers in the working situation; the nurses' reference groups, such as professional associations like ONA and the RNAO; and lastly, a nurse's own role image of what a nurse should be.

The CNO's mandate locates it as a rigid institution with evaluative criteria and goals for the nursing profession that influence how nurses think, feel, and act. At the unit level, the CNO is the organization that has the most influence because of its power to discipline nurses. The issue of the CNO's role in the disciplining of nurses allows for a structure that contributes to the dissatisfaction that staff nurses feel about their profession, as well as serving to contribute to the distance between the staff nurse and those in charge of nursing.

In the year 1997, 5,599 registered nurses did not renew their registration with the CNO. This is an increase of 138 percent compared to the 2,394 nurses who did not renew in 1994 (Political Election Platform, 1999, 9). This means that nurses who did not register are not working as nurses within the province of Ontario. This is not an old issue; registered nurses are taking early retirement, or are engaging in the 'casual' category.

In 2004, the CNO only reported those nurses who were not working, but did not state the numbers of those who did not renew their registration. The questions that our society must address are: "Why are nurses leaving the profession?" and "Who will be there to look after those who need nursing care?" According to an RNAO election-period advocacy document:

Registered nurses practicing in this [acute care hospital] are in extreme conflict, faced with the need to provide a much greater volume and intensity of care than they are able to deliver. Yet they remain responsible and accountable as professionals for practicing within the standards of the profession. As a result of this unsustainable situation, nurses are suffering from serious distress and burnout. (Political Election Platform 1999, 6)

The RNAO continued to publish statements that registered nurses are leaving the profession for opportunities that are "more acknowledged," "more respected," and "less emotionally painful."

At the unit level, there has been a de-skilling of the registered nurse through the placement of unregulated care providers. This stemmed from a mistaken belief that anyone with a little training could provide an adequate level of care to the patient, and that this would result in cost savings. Permanent and full-time positions have been reduced, and casual and part-time positions have increased (Political Election Platform 1999, 7).

At the unit level, the result was fragmented patient care, which left nurses feeling dissatisfied and frustrated. The unit provides a place for many staff nurses where they feel a sense of belonging within the hospital. Many staff nurses have informed me that they prefer eating in the unit lounge than going down to the hospital cafeteria. Staff nurses feel that they have more control within their patient care units, and can shape the culture of their unit. For the staff nurse, it is the unit in which they work that provides continuity, and community. Both at the professional level, and/or within the hospital, the larger community does not have an understanding of nurses' needs, and their desire to providing "good" patient care. Nurses view those outside of their own unit as "outsiders" and not part of their team. Even the ONA is not seen as doing all that is best for them. This attitude leaves staff nurses isolated at the unit level, and lacking participation and influence.

The Ministry of Health (MoH)

The MoH interacts with all the associations mentioned above and is a major player in that it sets standards and governs nurses through the Health Care and Hospital Acts it passes that overall create the structures, culture, and behaviour within the health care system. The work environment created through the Acts, however, is more complex than that created by government policies in that the organizations mentioned above are not micro-managed by the government. My argument is that the Ontario government, through laws and funding, influences work environments. Health care budgets, for example, are assigned to hospitals but are not micro-managed by the government. This gives hospitals control over how they use the dollars allocated to them. The government relies on nursing leaders and experts for advice on changes to policy that effect patient care and nurses. The strategies that nursing leaders take to government has implications for the staff nurse, including, for example, the educational standards for entry-level to the profession.

Most often, staff nurses, in spite of being at the forefront of the action, are distant from the decision-making process, and have not empowered themselves through the ONA. Indeed, staff nurses are "the centre" of the action because they are the individuals closest to the patient, and provide most of the treatments needed at the bedside, twenty-four hours a day. It is the nurse who first responds to a critical incident that occurs when a patient is in the hospital, and who provides information to the patient's physician. Although the nurses' care giving is constantly displaced by less skilled workers, it is the registered nurse who is responsible for the care that occurs on the unit.

In 1999, in order to strengthen patient care, the MoH invested $325 million in hospitals (Ontario, Ministry of Health 1999) by adding 1,400 nurses to wards, and another 440 to the emergency rooms. This increase in dollars was meant to relieve the workload of nurses, and to restore nursing services in the entire province. Staff nurses were under-represented on the Task Force, for the profession of nursing as a whole was under represented. Minority women were also under-represented, when the MoH was investigating the supply and demand of nurses in Ontario. Without attending to the voices of minority nurses—it is as if the MoH thinks that there is equity within the profession, and so does not need to seek out those who are from the margins.

This oversight makes the information that the MoH received one-sided—or top-sided. The inability of the Harris government to understand the concerns of ethnic minorities (who are becoming a majority within Toronto and the Greater Toronto Area [GTA]) can be seen in the way in which the Ontario government's Nursing Task Force reached out to stake holders. The report did not mention the racism (Das Gupta 1996; Collins et al. 1999) that ethnic minority nurses experience, although it was an issue that was discussed by scholars prior to the setting up of this Nursing Task Force.

When reviewing the demographics of nursing provided by the CNO to the government, the Task Force did not consider the ratio of Canadian graduates to immigrant nurses; such attention would have helped them understand the percentage of immigrant RNs within the nursing population, and that there might be problems for immigrant nurses in accessing the profession.

An area of importance in nursing research in 1999 was the "Quality of Nursing Worklife Research Unit" at the University of Toronto and McMaster University. The government of Ontario had provided funds for research. Once again, it is the elites within the profession who come from the dominant group that have access to these funds. The main interest of the Quality of Nursing Worklife Research Unit can be seen in its production of papers concerning nursing workload, nursing interventions, performance management, and restructuring; less visible is staff nurse job satisfaction. Also absent in the research is a discussion of racism, abuse, and harassment within the profession. Given the percentage of minority nurses within the profession, the lack of funds directed to research on topics such as racism shows a lack of understanding of the issues that face nursing today.

Understanding the Structure of Nursing

The RNAO, ONA, CNO, OHA, and MoH are not only influencing the profession of nursing, but also fight for public opinion in the changing face of health care, as public perception is vital in the restructuring of the health care system. In this kind of environment, conflict inevitably occurs among the organizations, which is then played out in public from time to time. This structure is complicated, with different partnerships on different occasions in an on-going jostle for power to have their ideas and goals influence the path that nursing should take.

Between the RNAO and the ONA, there is an additional fight to be the leader representing nurses rather than an alliance in order to speak for professional nursing. The RNAO views itself as the professional association representing 13,000 registered nurses throughout the health care spectrum, and the Ontario Nurses Association as the union representing 50,000. Since the ONA represents fifty-eight per cent of nurses registered in Ontario, it has the power in plain numbers to influence and strengthen the profession. With only fifteen per cent of registered nurses belonging to the RNAO, this organization's view of itself as the professional association while the ONA is a trade union must be viewed in the historical context of when the RNAO did not wish to be the bargaining unit for nurses. In Canada, most nursing associations are also the bargaining unit. The ONA, because of the number of nurses who are members, has more authority to speak on behalf of nurses; however, the MoH and the media still address their questions initially to the RNAO when nursing issues are areas of concern. When speaking for the registered nurse, the RNAO would only increase the association's power by collaborating with the ONA. Many nurses have chosen not to join the RNAO, but have joined the ONA, whose activity has improved the economic status and work environments of practicing nurses throughout Ontario. ONA has a role to improve the work environment for racialised nurses and be open to the views that they are still white at the top like the RNAO and the CNO.

The ONA views itself not only as a union, but also as a professional organization that provides ongoing education to its membership. In an interview, nurses informed me of what occurred regarding the two organizations:

> During our recent organization for nurses to join ONA, we saw the president of RNAO come out to the hospital and speak to the nurses regarding the benefits of joining the RNAO at the very time ONA was organizing the staff nurses, disregarding the fact that they do not have a mandate to involve themselves in labour relations and collective bargaining issues for staff nurses. (interview CO# 5)

As there is a networking link between the management nurses (who are OHA members) and the RNAO, an issue of unionized registered nurses (OHA members) who have been terminated due to cutbacks by hospital administration poses a question "of what good is the RNAO is to staff nurses?" The power of the RNAO has not decreased on account of a lowering membership base; the power of ONA has not increased on account of its large membership. The power struggle over who speaks for the registered nurse exists when both organizations want to deal independently with

83

the issues facing nursing, with little or no collaboration between them. It is time that the two organizations be merged in order that nurses have one voice speaking for them. This means that other unions such as CUPE should no longer represent the registered nurse. The OMA represents all doctors in Ontario. Like physicians, registered nurses need to have one organization representing them within the health care system and the ministry. Otherwise the situation leaves the OHA with the opportunity to divide and conquer the staff nurse body in its dealings with the MoH.

Although the ONA sits at the bargaining table for the staff nurse, the type of individual who nurses at the bedside is still the responsibility of nursing management within a hospital. If management chooses to replace the registered nurse with a health care aid, neither the CNO nor the ONA have a voice in the decision; the MoH also does not come into the decision-making process at this level. These decisions are made by a small group of nursing managers and are approved by hospital administration. The clash of perspectives and separate work relationships place management and staff in potential conflict with each other. In a discussion with her peers, and myself a staff nurse voiced the following:

> *These people* with their bureaucratic administration and authoritarian leadership which they deny. What it does to people at the staff level, they take you out of yourself, like control of your life. They tell you something you know is not true. They are not interested in the staff's welfare, they do not want you to take care of yourself. You do not want to anger them towards you. You can't talk back. You have to do what they want and not use your commonsense. If you do what you believe in and stand for your principles it can be a problem. They want you to behave they way they want. Either a little mouse or criticize them and be combative. (N.B., staff nurse, 1996, emphasis in the original)

The nurses in the group did not disagree with this comment; indeed, they added stories of how they viewed the power and the authority which administration has over the staff, which ONA can hold in check through the grievance process. It is through the process built in through collective bargaining that the ONA has authority and power to make sure that nurses are given due process and that nursing management and the hospital administration provide compensation when downsizing staff. Staff nurses expressed the view that without the ONA, they would be treated poorly by hospitals, both in terms of wages and in problem resolution with management.

Organized nursing through the RNAO and ONA also sets forth the values that guide the profession. These values do not conflict with the standards of the CNO. Along with the CNO's standards of practice, the ONA helps provide a basic standard in order that these expectations are somewhat the same in each hospital through bargaining contracts province-wide. The RNAO does, however, take positions on educational requirements (April 1996, 1999) for entry and the role of the registered nurse (September 1994); this is done in order to make changes that the elites within the profession view as important to the ongoing professionalization of nursing. Once again, the ONA and the RNAO have different agendas around the same issue, and they try and influence the CNO individually. This type of behaviour weakens the collaboration process.

It must be stated that nursing has not agreed on a model or theory to evaluate their practice within acute-care settings. At times nursing managers they use Benner (1982) to develop a frame of reference. This model goes from novice to expert. Benner argues that a competent and proficient nurse will not approach or solve a clinical situation in the same way each time it is encountered. The push to define and provide career ladders within clinical nursing has been difficult to standardize, and nursing has been struggling with issues around experience and education. Clinical practice is complex and does not provide for the creation of a smooth framework.

I have heard senior nurses state that "nurses have autonomy through the RHPA, an Act that makes nurses accountable and responsible for their practice." As discussed above, these are standards of care relatively independent of physicians, administrators, and other professionals. The CNO has provided standards of practice that gave a measure of autonomy needed for the staff nurse to practice as a nurse. Trying to influence the CNO's requirements for entry, the RNAO in its discussion paper calls for a baccalaureate degree in nursing as the educational requirement for entry into the RN profession (RNAO, April 1996, 1999). The ONA has many members who have been educated in the college system, and therefore has not addressed this issue in a public manner. All three nursing organization have agreed that the entry level for a RN in 2005 be a baccalaureate degree and have nursing schools and the college level link with universities. This has enabled students enrolling in 2004 at the college level to complete a baccalaureate degree, and this was one issue in which the RNAO, CNO, and ONA spoke out in one voice. Soon thereafter, each organization issued their own statements as to how the health system should be restructured when the Ontario government wanted to close hospitals. This makes for conflicting messages on the part of those who speak out for nursing, but at times also benefits the MoH in that the Ministry can legitimate its position by citing the organization of its choice on each issue concerning nurses. This structure of relations makes for the profession of nursing a weakened structure wherein decisions are made according to each organization's own agenda, yet ultimately at the mercy of outside forces. The MoH with its Task Force on Nursing (September 1998) worked with all four organizations to analyse nursing utilization and retention, however, there is a nursing shortage within acute care. Perhaps staff nurses through their association need to take the lead role in addressing why this is occurring and not leave it to those in management and research to speak out on their behalf.

Examining the Structure

We see that all four organizations have an interest in the role of the registered nurse. The CNO represents the public interest, the OHA the institution, the RNAO represents the professional view, and the ONA union represents the staff nurse group. All four parts make up "the structure" in which decisions about the profession of nursing is made; this constitutes the professional structure. For the staff nurse, however, the strongest part of this structure in relationship to the role of the professional nurse is the CNO. This is due to the fact that the CNO is backed by core legislation that establishes the governing framework for nursing in the province, which helps it to define the scope of practice for nursing. The CNO is not linked to any other of the parts within this structure and has eighteen public members appointed to the Council by the provincial government. The CNO is the only organization that sets standards of nursing practice and professional behaviour, which identify expectations for providing nursing care that all registered nurses must follow. Because the CNO protects the public by looking into complaints about the practice of nurses, it is a major provider to the nursing profession's belief system and behaviour, a topic that will be discussed in another chapter. All other organizations are influenced by the CNO's standards in addressing expectation of the role of the registered nurse. The MoH, however, has economic power as it is the sole financial agency to all the players within the structure. Hospitals receive their global budgets from the MoH and have economic micro-control over the role of the staff nurse.

In examining the four organizations and their roles within this professional structure, we find four organizations that lack co-ordination between them, although they all articulate the need for a high-quality health care system. With four competing roles, rather than completing each other and working together as one structure, we see the four as dividing the issues as to best meet their own agendas. The exercise of power has been discussed with three out of the four structures having power to affect direct changes to the profession.

There is a formal hierarchy of authority within this system, with the CNO at the top when it comes to the role of the registered nurse. It sets the tone for how the nurse behaves, however, in terms of hospital culture and workplace, the hospital and through it the OHA is at the top. Although both the CNO and the OHA want to ensure high-quality health care for the people of Ontario, they lack direct decision-making authority over what constitutes safe nursing care, including patient-staff ratios. The CNO does not assist the OHA in defining the evolving role of hospitals within a restructured system, nor does the OHA in its formal role assist the CNO when they deal with standards for nursing registration. The lack of an established process whereby the ONA and the RNAO, the two nursing major stakeholders, can discuss and develop policy for the profession, shows a professional structure that does not foster a participatory and consensus-building environment. The ONA for one views the CNO as "not the registered nurse's friend." The College wishes to be fair to the membership, while balancing this with public protection. The ONA does not see this balance, and also views the CNO as silent on issues that affect nurses in acute care when standards of practice. The CNO wants input into the health care system and calls for unity (*Communiqué* 1997a, 5), as it views splinters as weakening "ourselves." Instead, each organization tries its best to speak out as to what they think the profession of nursing should or should not be doing. If real collaboration occurred, the relationship between the two organizations would help the nurse.

Joint ventures between the RNAO and the ONA around political strategies that strengthen the role of the profession within the health care system, both in the institutional and non-institutional context, have not been an ongoing strategy. There is little detectable demonstration of collaboration between these organizations when they publicize the values of the nursing profession. While gathering the data for researching collegiality, I was informed that due to the competition in representing nurses, the RNAO had intervened when the ONA was trying to organize registered nurses at a particular hospital. I was also made aware that a strain in relationship occurred with a formal notification from the ONA requesting a cooling-off period away from the RNAO, and the ONA stopped working with them on projects concerning nursing issues (M.P., interview, 1998). This struggle hurts the staff nurses, as these organizations that speak for them are in conflict with each other over their relative power, attitudes, and importance. In my review of the two organizations, the RNAO serves the management and educational group of nurses far more than the staff nurse group. The RNAO lacks the authority to speak for the staff nurse due to the fact that it is closely allied with the administrative views held by hospitals and universities. The ONA is the organization that has the interest of the staff nurse at heart and does focus its resources on the needs and wishes of its membership. Until the RNAO and the ONA engage in a collaborative effort to produce a united front for the profession, the cause of nursing will suffer. To unite the RNAO and ONA would require a focus beyond the short-term rewards and a search for success over the long term. In all other provinces in Canada, there are not two separate organizations for nursing as there are in Ontario; nurses are represented by one nursing organization for both their professional and labour concerns.

All three nursing organizations—the ONA, the RNAO, and the CNO—do not strategically communicate the value of nursing to legislators, the media, and other influential structures within health care. Each nursing organization markets its own view and at times does so at the expense of the other. The role of the nurse within the hospital, and the education entry level for the registered nurse, were and are issues that these organizations could have collaborated on; however, the conflict arising from this issue has been lingering since I was a student nurse. Thirty years later, the debate continues. When strategies should be discussed, attention is paid instead to the agendas of each organization. For the gap to be bridged there has to be power sharing and open communication among the players within the structure. Since decisions are based on economic values rather than the profession of nursing as restructuring occurs, the decisions effecting nursing are occurring with very little input from the ONA, the CNO, and the RNAO.

In Ontario, power and politics in nursing are mainly embedded in economics, the legal system, and with the government. Both the ONA and the RNAO have discovered how politics and power are linked, and both are working individually to exert influence such that that they are the primary speakers for the nursing profession within Ontario. The current climate in the structure is not one of co-operation in decision-making, rather, the essential characteristics are power struggles, drawing public attention to one's views, and influencing policy makers. At bottom, the formation of power alliances with each other has not been formalized among the nursing groups, although an attempt has been made by the RNAO to collaborate with both the OMA and the ONA over nursing care issues. The question of leaving ONA out of the loop when working with physicians leads me to argue that the RNAO is positioning itself to gain power and be the voice of the nursing profession. Although not happy with the MoH, the OMA through the JPPC (or any new arm of the MoH) has input into the decision-making process. These alliances, however, are not in the interest of the staff nurses (as they are not part of the JPPC) but in the interest of the existing power brokers—MoH, OMA, and the OHA—within the health system. Physicians have historically more power than nurses and because of the many unions and associations representing nurses; their voice is diluted—which again dis-empowers them as women. We also know that white women have more power than racialised women in nursing. Where are their voices?

This structure of relations wherein decisions are made about the profession is one which reflects the culture of the government and its decision-making behaviour. The behaviour of the MoH as discussed in this chapter shows that it does not view nursing as a profession, as it does with medicine. The MoH usually approaches one organization in dealing with nurses, while neglecting to bring the four organizations together in order to discuss patient-staff ratios, the work environment, and standards for entry and practice. Therefore, the conflict that occurs between these organizations provides a professional structure wherein staff nurses feel left out and powerless as changes occur around them. The MoH in its decision-making structure has different policy silos that are not interactive but competitive in maintaining their individual and with it the funds and resources that each silo controls within the health care system. This behaviour, of fighting for power rather than of power sharing, trickles down to the organizations that compete for resources to maintain their agencies. Hospitals in Ontario use the most resources and have the most funding; therefore, they have the most power when compared with other institutions in the health care system. Since MoH controls the resources that fund nursing care, they use this economic power when addressing issues concerning the profession of nursing and how nurses are treated within the health care system. Until the MoH, when discussing the nursing profession, views all organizations that employ, educate, register, and represent nursing as one entity, nurses will have competing interests, and competing representation.

With the significant changes that have occurred and continue to occur in the financing of health care in Ontario, public expectations of health care delivery have correspondingly changed. Each new government brings forward policies on which they campaigned. Given that the delivery of health care is a major concern of Canadians, each new government tries to carry out some form of health care reform. As organizations within the structure of the profession of nursing are experiencing increasing pressure to implement change, the views expressed by the four organizations discussed here have a substantial impact on the direction that the nursing profession takes.

Often, through media communications, the philosophy, values, and policies of hospitals are transferred as health care values to the general public. Using tax dollars, hospitals send out newsletters to the public addressing health care issues and the hospital's 'good news' items. Most hospitals do not have a Vice President of Nursing; some have Chief Officers of Nursing, whose mandate is to look at nursing within their hospitals, while the managing of nursing care is under other administration personal. This gives hospital administrators and the OHA an advantage over organizations such as the ONA and staff nurses.

The public only understands what they view at the bedside, and thus, the politics underlying how decisions are made concerning nursing care is not their focus. In addition, given that they are discussed in committee meetings and in Boardrooms, this information is not available to the general public. The employee does not have the ability to go to the media as a whistle-blower, while hospitals can speak to the media through their Public Relations Officers. When an incident occurs, it is the official version that is placed on record.

In analysing the four organizations, it must be noted that conflict and tension arise when the value system of a particular organization creates demands. or views its agenda as the more important one for nurses. Unless the MoH views the ONA is as important for the health care system, staff nurses will not have real input into the changing face of health care, in direct planning for better patient care, or how dollars are, as one respondent comments: "wasted in hospital."

The current structure continues to hamper the staff nurses' quest for acceptance as full 'players' within the health care system. In terms of professional autonomy, power is an essential element in the professionalization process. In order to increase its power, the ONA should become more politically active, so that it could emerge as a powerful political force. Until the ONA sits at the table as does the OMA in discussions with the JPPC, the current environment, which is dominated by hospitals and the medical profession, will continue to influence the culture of the nursing profession, and the structure described in this chapter. The struggles within the structure cause the linkages that have to be addressed to become lost. In addition, the framework within which system alliances can occur gets buried. No structure can be sustained if the parts act at cross-purposes with each other. As will be discussed in the next chapter, these four organizations lack alliances with one another, which has implications for the culture of nursing collegiality.

This structure provides an environment for the inter-group conflict that exists between the staff nurses and the academic and administrative nurse leaders within the nursing profession. These conflicts were primarily surrounding patient-staff ratios, and non-professional caregivers. The staff nurses hold the view that all registered nurses are professional, no matter what type of school they graduate from, while the leadership within the profession push for a baccalaureate degree.

Of course, the goal of nursing education is to socialize the individual into acquiring a philosophy of nursing and mastering treatment tasks. Nursing faculties in academia provide socialization through which the education professional controls the production of future nurses, imprinting on them the tenets of the 'ideal type' of nurse. The "ideal nurse is trained in a university environment" debate angers those nurses trained in hospitals and colleges. The conflict arises from the perception that university-trained nurses are professional nurses whose education preparation is different from those trained in colleges and hospitals. Some scholars do not view these nurses as professional (Kramer 1974; Chitty 1997). The faculty role provides a platform where a nurse on faculty can lecture and write about what constitutes the professional nurse (Moloney 1992), or the collegial nurse (Styles 1982), and can provide a description of the behaviours expected of registered nurses.

Nurses who wish to become part of the leadership in nursing may choose to inculcate and cultivate the standards of 'the ideal'. Those individuals who are committed to working as a staff nurse may not follow the leadership or accept their values since they do not meet their own standards of the meaning of nursing work. The consequences of the conflict between the nursing leadership (Academic Nursing, Clinical Educators, Nursing Administrators) through its organ, the RNAO, and the staff nurse group through the ONA, creates a source of conflict between the ONA and the RNAO *as organizations*, and between management nurses and staff nurses. At the same time, through these competing views on professionalization between the staff nurses within their organization, the ONA, can increase their own membership cohesion. There is a price to be paid for the current competition and power struggle that is occurring within the profession of nursing. I am of the opinion that the conflict between these two groups influences the culture of nursing, and thus collegial behaviours. For social justice to occur within nursing, the structures need to examine systemic oppressions, systemic racism, and the leadership that allows it to occur.

Notes

1   The educational arm, such as the University of Toronto's nursing faculty, is not viewed as part of the structure for this research due to the fact that once a student leaves the educational institution, it no longer controls the nursing life of the nurse and it does not have a part in the day-to-day organizational life of the staff nurse.

2   Such symbols have mostly disappeared, as most nurses today do not believe that nursing is about what they wear, but what they do.

3   In later chapters, I will further describe and analyse this issue in my discussion of culture and behaviour.

Chapter Four

The Production of Professional Culture

Cultural considerations serve to determine the quality and nature of the relationships that occur between the actors involved. In the last chapter, four organizations were discussed in terms of their interconnectedness as a structure that fits together in a set pattern revolving around relations of power. The analysis in this chapter points both to the *culture* that arises from the interactions that have occurred over time, as well as recent interactions.

As the detailed discussion of the structure revealed, the impact on the staff nurse group on the culture of the profession more generally, is such that individual organizations within the structure are uneven in terms of power and influence. Race and class become important variables of exploitation and abuse within the culture of nursing. Professionalism as a project in nursing led to a cultural shift from nursing as devalued women's work to the patriarchal equation of nursing and cultural identity of the professional nurse. Constructions of the "ideal" nurse as representative of this cultural change ensured that certain classes of women would perform certain types of labour. Educated white middle-class women who construct elaborate rules are now the elite representing nursing within the Canadian health care system. Working-class, and racialised women were not their concern, and they continued to use them as cheap labour, caring for patients as "personal assistants." The limits in the education of this group of care-givers promote certain types of labour that the elites do not view as 'nursing proper'.

Again, as nursing culture changes, many issues such as racism within nursing remain unresolved. Attempts are made to understand sexuality, racism, disability, and to promote social justice, as articulated through nursing standards. Repressive practices are still, however, reported within the profession (Das Gupta 2005; Hagey et al. 2002, 2005; Jacobs 2000, 2002, 2006).

The hospital environment in which nursing work occurs provides values and norms about work and about the interactions that take place there. These interactions produce an *organizational culture* within each hospital. Nursing culture also is predicated upon the interplay of social, economic, and political factors that influences the internal hospital environment. Thus, the effects of unit and hospital closures on the working environment (van der Wal et al. 1998) had psychological impacts and changed the culture of the environment as staff were moved from unit to unit or were laid off; employees were not likely to smile, and events were related in a negative rather than a positive manner; staff took longer breaks; and things went missing from the hospital. Those affected lacked motivation and exhibited a "don't care" attitude towards both themselves and others. In this environment, patriarchal discourses, white privilege, and racism are hidden within the changes that are taking place. Clearly, such a context affects collegiality.

As discussed in the last chapter, formal organizations constitute the institutionalized environment wherein the organizational culture of the nursing profession develops. At the staff nurse level, the culture *per se* is evaluated by staff nurses, and can be rejected or accepted, thus nurses do exercise some large measure of 'agency' in their environment. As a group, staff nurses also produce norms and values at the unit level that produce a *sub*culture that is particular to the specific unit. As such, there can be several different subcultures within the one organization. Elements of the macro-level culture can, however, be experienced in every subculture.

As the list of influences is potentially open-ended, I have narrowed it to the definition of the culture that arises from the organized structure of professions and collegiality as described by Bess: "Culture exists not in physical, palpable form, but as a collection of ideas about behaviours that exists in the minds of organizational workers" (1988, 92). Another way of understanding the culture of nursing is by viewing the profession through the lens of *caring*, as nursing culture was built on the values of caring and devotion, as epitomized by the Nightingale Pledge (see the introduction).

In Turner's view, a subculture is a distinctive set of meanings shared by a specified group, who ensure that newcomers undergo a particular process of learning or socialization that reproduces past elements (Turner 1977). It is assumed that the collection of ideas about nursing behaviour has come from the institutional level "top down," and not from the grassroots up—from the very origin of the profession. The ideas about behaviour originate in professional standards and policies, and when accepted by student nurses become the "idea" of the nurse.

As with any participants in a group, nurses must know the culture in order to be fully functioning members who can decode cultural meaning, and shape this into efficient guides to everyday behaviour. In order to

94

decode the meanings within the profession and within the hospital, staff nurses must be aware of the formal culture of the profession, as well as the culture of the particular hospital in which they work. Again, the staff nurse group within the hospital is not passive in absorbing the hospital or professional culture. They also react to behaviours that occur within the organization, disagreeing and opposing some, while upholding those behavioural issues with which they are in agreement, within the standards of their profession. At times, staff nurses are silent, as if acquiescing to the changes that are taking place. This does not necessarily mean an acceptance of such changes, but rather can indicate a "don't care" attitude, which is a withdrawal of interaction.

Relations with other health care workers also play a part in providing values and behaviours to the group. Morgan (1986) points out that one way of appreciating the nature of culture is to observe the day-to-day functioning of a group or organization to which one belongs. This point of view ties in with my experiences, and observations as a nurse, and adds another dimension to the understanding of the culture of the profession of nursing. Nursing culture is more than the issue of professionalization; it is also the exploration of the complexities of working women's consciousness within a predominately female profession. Therefore, culture provides for the environment wherein nurses judge the observable behaviour of the other. The insight gained from being female, from their education, and their understanding of what inhabiting the margins is about, is both a strength and a limitation for objective judgement.

In addition, nursing work, which is women's work, is devalued due to old double-standards, as well as by messages communicated to the public that were in the interest of the powerful—usually men (Armstrong and Armstrong 1990). Thus, this culture consists of the norms and values passed down since Nightingale; collected values from the professional structure which are passed along to staff nurses through written instructions, and verbal communication; the observable behaviour of nurses which student nurses emulate based on the "nursing role;" and the construction of gender identities, as well as constructs of ethno-racial identities.

Many aspects of this culture are embedded in the everyday practice of caring and providing treatment for patients. Nurses transmit their subcultural knowledge by word of mouth, and by demonstration (Wolf 1988, 68). Nursing symbols and rituals, such as the capping ceremony, which has been discarded, convey significant information about the profession's culture. There are several reasons why caps and uniforms began to disappear in the 1970s. As nursing wanted to become more professionalized, nurses began to identify more with doctors and other professionals who wore no uniform; the standard uniforms differentiated them into a pink ghetto. Wolf (1988) states that these rituals enable nurses to carry out caring activities for patients who are acutely or chronically ill, old, and dying. Although some researchers view nursing rituals as wasting time (Huttmann 1985), nursing rituals helped nurses to reaffirm some of the beliefs and values of nursing, such as doing good, and avoiding harm.

Understanding nursing culture is also to understand nurses within the context of their relationships with other health care providers, patients, and her/his significant others. This environment also includes issues of abuse, harassment, racism, and oppression. As one explores the rationale for these aspects of the workplace culture, we find that they are similar to those issues that women and minorities confront within the larger society. Nursing culture is also tied into other provincial health care and re-organizational issues of the health care system, some of which were discussed in the previous chapter (and see Ross 1961; Corwin 1961; Taves, Corwin, and Hass 1963; Kramer 1968; Ashley 1976; Chaska 1978; Muff 1982; Armstrong 1984; Campbell 1988; Reverby 1987; Grow 1991; Chaska 1992; Jacobs 2000, 2002; Hagey and MacKay 2000; Hagey et al. 2001).

Constructing the Culture of Nursing Within a Jurisdiction

Nurse leaders within the RNAO, the CNO, and those within university networks form an "old girls" club that dominates the direction and the vision of nursing and helps set the career path for nurses whom they mentor. Nurse leaders make an effort to involve themselves within the RNAO and the CNO. They influence changes that take place concerning clinical issues, codes of ethics, and policies for practice. The participation in the RNAO and the CNO at the staff level is more limited, thereby making nursing culture at this level more about elite participation through the latter's heavy involvement in the nursing hierarchy. Nursing cultures are also bureaucratized through committee structures. Participants within this hierarchy take recommended changes back to their hospitals where they attempt to implement them. Staff nurses, in their discussions with me concerning their roles, were more interested in changing their immediate environment. For staff nurses to attend meetings at the RNAO or ONA is to

structural obstacles that prevent nurses at lower levels to be heard go beyond their institution or workplace, and to interact at a professional level that takes time away from family life and that does not address their needs. Shift work was another reason for the lack of time and energy to participate outside working hours in their professional organizations. Staff nurses could not attend meetings when they worked two weeks on day and two weeks of an evening or night shift. Staff nurses are marginalized and do not see how the margins can shift the centre composed of nurses in management and academia. I would conclude from my observations, that nurses in management and education that need to network with colleagues at the RNAO and CNO are supported in doing so. They are provided with the flextime and the means to extend beyond the hospital or university to participate in professional organizations and activities. On the other hand, it is difficult for staff nurses to receive the same considerations, thereby precluding them from the same level of participation. Thus, while they remain hostile about their overall situation, yet by not participating, they perpetuate the current culture.

The CNO, ONA, and the RNAO contribute to the regulations and standards surrounding professionalism and collegial behaviour. Rules and regulations are often created at the professional or organizational level and can be invoked as part of a power play by nurse managers over the staff nurse, providing for a bureaucratic decision-making process to regulate behaviours that is the location where experts exert power over the staff nurse group. Staff nurses rarely report on management's deleterious behaviours. Standards in nursing are therefore the tools of the elite within the profession.

One of the key elements of any profession is the expert knowledge that defines it. Theories of nursing, the development of which began around 1960 (Bullough and Bullough 1994), are hardly adequate as "expert knowledge". They function as *ideologies* and are all-pervasive within the culture of the nursing profession; they serve as the basis of a framework for nursing practice and are tied to the 'professionalization' of nursing. Clearly, when staff nurses are providing care to their patients, it does not matter to them if a theory relates to or governs their practice. What matters to them is that their work environments and that the standards, policies, and values for encounters with peers and patients be understood by members of the health care team. One nurse commented thus:

> I enjoy reading the different theories in nursing. My main complaint is when... my manager tries to push her chosen theory... it does not help my work. (D.L., staff nurse medicine, 1996)

> We are so short staffed and they [management] can sit and talk about picking a theory so that we will be more professional. Theory is fine, but it does not provide better care for my patients. Usually, it makes more paper work, or a change in how we chart—until they get on to their next bandwagon. Don't get me wrong, I like to expand my nursing knowledge but what is happening is one change after another for the sake of some one in management who has a project at university or a new idea...." (E.D., staff nurse, Out Patient Department, 1995)

This respondent's comments helps to point out that if the leadership transplants ideology as a substitute for a theoretical framework, it becomes the embodiment of social relations and the culture of work—something that the staff nurse is not necessarily willing to embrace. This is understandable if we note that harassment of "the other" because of differences of ideology becomes an acceptable form of behaviour on the part of the experts in nursing theories. The staff nurse feels as if the "experts" in nursing theories are seeking to make them into obedient subjects who yield to their authority.

I use the term "other," to point to the way dominant groups act in achieving their goals. Perceptions are filtered through cultural locations, and culture acts as a shield that legitimizes inequalities. Rules that exist to guide activities can also be used to block and control activities within a profession. Staff nurses experience blocking and control as harassment when they reject and/or implement other ways of understanding nursing approaches.

Nursing educators in university also play an important part in nursing identity by formulating theoretical constructs (Johnson 1958; King 1981; Roy 1983; Orem 1985) for nursing practice. Theorist such as Johnson, King, Roy and Orem provide structure and/or understanding to the actions of nursing through their theories on nursing. Johnson (1958), the first nursing theorist, was however, influenced by sociologists; and Neuman (1982), like other early nursing theorists, draws directly from general systems theory. Nursing theories such as Roy's theory of adaptation (1983), are regarded by nurse managers and nursing leaders in many hospitals as a basis for nursing practice.

Nurse administrators use nursing theories as the culture of practice, and expect it to promote certain values within the nursing department, or division of their institution. In my observations, although all nurses are aware of nursing theory as it is a part of their curriculum in both college and university programmes, nursing theory has not been widely accepted by the staff nurse as a process for providing patient care. It is accepted that students will use nursing theories to help them in their clinical practice within hospitals, and that through educational processes a culture of nursing will be promoted. As discussed later, experienced staff nurses view those coming into the profession with BSN degrees as having only theory, and not knowing how to perform required practical tasks.

Staff nurses, by their lack of participation in the professional structures and their lack of empowerment, have given nursing leaders participating in professional structures an important dimension of power over them. This lack of participation by staff nurses has entrenched the hierarchy of nursing and allowed the leadership the major role in shaping the values that guide the profession. — blaming the victim?

Through the ONA staff nurses can participate by voting in their leadership that negotiates collective agreements with hospitals, and that attempts to restore a sense of balance for the staff nurse. In 2003, however, during the last election of the organisation's president, only a minority of members participated in electing their leader. The lack of participation in union elections can be seen as a message that staff nurses do not view their organizations as speaking in their best interest. They may also not view those in leadership positions as contributing to their understanding and resolution of the problems they face as staff nurses.

Within the nursing profession, rituals are created during the educational period and sustained and passed on through hospital practice and myths is a reality of nursing discourse and attitudes. Rituals such as admitting a patient or laying out the dead are some examples. Rituals and symbols are often embedded not only in the formal structures that come out of the actions taken by the organizations—the OHA, the ONA, the CNO, the RNAO, as well as within the Universities' Nursing programs—but are also passed down from nurse to nurse as they work together within hospitals. "Nursing talk" occurs in the everyday life of the staff nurse and helps to shape ideas, values and rituals For example, how staff nurses in a specific unit start their shift is filled with ritual and is an area for further research.

Over the years, several feminists have noted that women's work around caring is devalued, and we need to pursue the question of how nurses are socialized to operate within patriarchal structures and patriarchal discourses of professionalism. Nursing hierarchy embraces the notions of professionalism operating with patriarchal structures of power without really focusing on advocating against the violent action of racism that is perpetrated against racialised nurses and racialised patients.

While many Euro-American feminists have looked at women's work and deconstructed patriarchal power, they have not focused the same lens on their white sisters and their use of power in a predominantly multi-racial work force. The use of cultural competencies to understand racism and limit its practice does not embrace new thinking (See for example: Das Gupta, 1966) but attempts to ignore the present escalation of racism within the nursing culture. The central focus of nursing is caring, yet eating their young, horizontal violence, and racism flourish in what I call a toxic professional nursing environment that is dominated by Eurocentric thinking.

Hospital culture more generally provides insight into the "autonomy" value that is part of the culture of nursing, and is also a value in 'professionhood'. Culture can also be understood through examining notions of the ideal nurse, the professional nurse, job promotions, and abuse and racism within the profession. One perspective that was voiced by staff nurses in response to the question "What makes a real nurse?" maintained that it is nurses who understand and embrace a culture in which caring, support, and respect are valued as a norm.

From the leadership's perspective, professionalism embraces values that involve an implicit assumption that increased education produces "the professional nurse", and enhances research-based practice. The culture of nursing is constructed from a Euro-American and Eurocentric perspectives, using old patriarchal structures, rather than anti-racist feminist discourse. This is, of course understandable, given that an anti-racism praxis is oppositional to white hegemony, and the attendant social, economic, and political interests.

Understanding the meaning of whiteness and the power and privilege of white skin, which is largely invisible to those who possess it (see, e.g., Puzan 2003), is also an important aspect of this thinking. Another dimension to anti-racism theory is a critique of liberalism, such as individualism, equal opportunity, colour blindness, education, and the focus on incremental change. How then do we construct the culture of collegiality?

The Culture of the "Ideal" Nurse

As the methods of the leadership changes, the construction of the "ideal" nurse becomes more regulated. Working as a nurse in Ontario for the past twenty-eight years, I have observed changes in what constituted this "ideal" nurse. These include an external image alteration, such as allowing nurses to wear coloured garments; and a change in the values and norms around both the behaviour, and the role of the nurse in health care.

As a student, I was informed that the "lighted lamp" from the Nightingale image was important, and that it "was service and not fame" that was the ideal. As part of the role of a "good nurse," nurses were to care for the sick, help each other, and not unionize; they could belong to an association if the wished. They did not have input into changes within the occupation, but instead concentrated on day-to-day activities. Today, it is professional standards, clinical practice, and the development and application of a body of knowledge that nursing researchers produce, and is adhered to by the "professional" nurse.

Nursing practice through nursing research is a value that is promoted at the leadership level, while staff nurses' values centre around knowledge, experience, and intuition—"gut intuition" has saved many patients lives. One interviewee commented thus:

> I had just made my hourly rounds and was at the desk talking to another nurse and I felt something. A feeling. I just walked straight to the bathroom and found this lady hanging from a pipe with a sheet. We cut her down and saved her life. It just came, this strange feeling that I had to check that room as I had just checked it. Boy.... (A.J., staff nurse, psychiatry, 1995)

> I was at the desk charting and I felt I had to go and check my patient in room... there was no need. He was okay and recovering nicely, but something inside of me said go and see Mr. X. When I got to the room, I saw he was short of breath and looked grey. If I had not gone in he would have died, as I had

to call a code. I find that my gut feelings, and not just the lab work have helped me with so many of my patients. Like just feeling someone is going to take a turn for the worse. I also find that family who have not visited a patient for weeks will come when we are in a middle of a code. That has happened so many times, it is like they know. The more experience I have, this gut feeling makes me go and check. At times nothing is wrong but I feel better for checking.... (M.P., interview 1995, staff nurse, medicine).

Experience and intuition are important aspects of the expected makeup of the ideal bedside nurse. Skills learned through experience compete with book knowledge, and attitudes are formed as to which is valued the more in a given situation. The debate brings with it an emphasis on professionalism, and on how it impacts the culture of the unit, the hospital, and the profession as a whole. The staff nurse is linked to her unit group, then to the nurses at large in the hospital, and then to the profession. The role relationship of the staff nurse involves more than one type of relationship, and depends on the situation, as well as the framework in which it occurs. This then means that the perception of the ideal nurse changes, depending on the role of the staff nurse, and the type of work in which she/he is engaged.

The culture of the current "ideal" nurse includes the notion of the upgrading of knowledge, or of "up-skilling". For example, the ideal nurse is considered to be someone who practices nursing care through a nursing theory model, and who uses nursing research to guide her or him. She/he must also have a BSN degree, and understands the *process* of nursing, rather than exhibiting a focus on single tasks. Although taught critical thinking, student nurses are still educated in a cookie-cutter type of model, in which "one size fits all".

The ideal nurse is also expected to take part in committee work, and update her/his education; yet most staff nurses have children, and are the primary caregivers. Staff nurses have stated that they do not have the time to stay after work, or go in on their days off for committee work. With cutbacks to staff, they also feel that they are overworked, and do not have time to attend educational sessions that occur within their hospitals. Staff nurses do stay current, however, by reading nursing journals, and they certainly agree with the importance of keeping their knowledge up to date. We find that when asked about reading journals, 10.9% of nurses rarely read nursing journals, compared to the 89.1% who update themselves by reading current nursing journals. Staff nurses are provided with nursing journals at the hospitals where they work; and they also receive a monthly newsletter from the CNO. Therefore, a culture of knowledge exists, and has become part of the nursing culture, whereas committee work, and university education are not viewed in the same manner.

For the staff nurse, the culture of the ideal nurse is centred on the care-giving aspects of nursing, and the values related to such care. Committee work that produces "rules and more paper," is looked upon as having less value than a meeting among peers to discuss the care of a patient. Although the physician is the person who writes orders, there are nursing care issues that lie outside of these orders. Discussions with physicians and other health professionals are important actions for the nurse as it is in this arena that the nurse advocates for her or his patient. For the staff nurse, the ideal nurse is one who does all she/he can for the patient and the family and assists her/his colleagues. The manager's view of the ideal nurse overlaps with the staff nurse's view in terms of respect and support for peers, advocacy for patients, and educating patients and families. The leadership/manager view of the ideal nurse is one who has far more undertakings outside working hours to help promote a culture of continuing education, and professional participation in organizations like the RNAO. This view has less significance with staff nurses, and so participation levels relate to the identification the individual has with the profession, and the level of direct involvement with patient care.

It seems clear that the closer the nurse is to the patient, the more involvement there is at the unit level. On the other hand, administrators have more involvement with research, and with working on nursing standards at the organizational level; this includes methods for valid measurement of nursing workload, and productivity/utilization. They are also concerned with understanding the staff nurse's relationship with the patient, other nurses, and with system outcomes (O'Brien-Pallas et. al. 2004).

The construction of the ideal nurse is critically related to a Euro-American view of nursing, and is related to the nature of socio-economic class. Nursing researchers (Lowe 2006; O'Brien-Pallas et. al. 2004; McGillis Hall 2003; Donner et al. 1994; Baumann and O'Brien-Pallas 1993) discuss creating work environments that foster nurses' mental and physical health, safety, security, and satisfaction, without looking into the behaviour of nurse managers described in this study. Racialised nurses', who are predominantly working class women, struggle within the nursing profession surfaces as "oppositional" to the progress in nursing. Nursing researchers' politics of professional building is linked to the ideal nurse, and a departure from the idealized vision of nursing. This has had negative consequences. My argument is that for staff nurses the ideal nurses has not been constructed with them in mind, nor has the intersections of race and class constituted part of nursing categorisation. Rather, the monolithic approach to the construction of this image grants it a privileged place that it does not deserve within a multicultural society.

The Professional Nurse as a Cultural Value

Currently, the ideal nurse is constructed as a professional (Jacobs 2006). Nurse leaders provide desirable standards and values (Styles 1982) irrespective of the views expressed by staff nurses or nurse managers outside the network. I have heard from nurse managers that the term "professional nurse" equates with higher education or a baccalaureate degree. What I recognized about professionalism is that it brings to the culture of nursing a value that is less about nursing care, and more about legitimate claims of nursing autonomy on the part of leaders within the profession. A profession must have some degree of autonomy. This autonomy provides the leadership with authority and control over the rank and file in the profession.

As discussed in earlier chapters, accountability is also a professional requirement, and nurses are expected to report those who have deviated from the standards of professional practice. This type of accountability is not part of the culture of physicians, or other professionals working in a hospital. From my discussions with staff nurses in Metro Toronto, professionalism for them is tied to job content and providing patient care. They are aware, however, that there is a push to replace staff nurses who do not have degrees with those who have BSN degrees. This push produces fear and anger in many nurses who are hospital or college trained. Education then becomes a divider, rather than an element for the provision of knowledge and skills for better patient care. Two staff nurses offer their views on this issue:

> They hired this BSN nurse and after orientation she came to
> work one evening with me. When I asked her to start an IV
> for a patient, she told me she would not do it. After a while

she came and asked me how to give an injection, as she had not done one before. She was very quiet and scared but did not know how to do any practical work. They know their theory of how to but have no skills to do what they need to do. I helped her but management values these unskilled nurses more than us and our knowledge. (S.V., maternal-child care division, 1996)

I find that University trained nurses know their process and can talk about what the book states. They have very little training and cannot see the patient in trouble when they first come out of school. A patient was going into a code and this nurse came to me and was very anxious. We provide professional care and know our work. At the bedside if you do not know what you are doing the patient can die. I have a gut feeling that something can go wrong and you cannot learn this from books, only through time with patients and clinical experience during training like we had. Now nurses get very little hours at the bedside. (E.S., surgery, 1996)

These two views on the BSN and professionalism are samples of what staff nurses verbalise as a problem around management's attitude towards higher education. There are also differences between the educational programs that train nurses, and this places one type of educational program above another. Staff nurses who do not have BScN degrees do not, however, acknowledge these differences, and instead, see their training as equal, or even superior. They view themselves as professionals, and consider nurses who graduated from university programmes as "book trained", and with little experience at the bedside. They resent their lack of experience in patient care. Comments on "attitudes of feeling superior" provide diploma nurses with an argument that she or he used to limit discussions and understanding between the two types of training.

My observations of BSN nurses in action is that those who work at the bedside have an inclusive attitude, while those in management, or those who aspire to have leadership roles are far more elitist. Elements of educational values, when advanced into the issue of who or what is a professional nurse, brings with it a devaluing of the strengths that exist in both the university and the diploma/hospital schools of nursing. All nurses share the value of the professional nurse; it is the push for nursing degrees that is the root cause of the current conflict in this regard. The competing views about who is a professional nurse thus create conflict, rather than collegial co-operation among staff nurses.

The inter-group conflict regarding education was created between the group of staff nurses and the leaders within the nursing profession when they embarked on a labelling system. The latter labelled some nurses as "technical" registered nurses, and others who are university graduates as "registered nurses". This latter group they considered to be the "professional" nurses.

The label "technical nurses" emphasises the lower status that nursing leadership places on those nurses trained in hospitals and colleges. These nurses work as bedside nurses, and are the ones with whom the public comes into contact (Chitty 1997). This debate angers those nurses trained in hospitals and colleges, for in their view, all registered nurses are professional, no matter what type of school they attended.

Professional advancement is one of the main foci of the professional nurse (Chitty 1997). Many staff nurses view themselves as professional, not technical nurses; they thus do not place value on the labels provided by those in nursing leadership positions. For those not trained in universities, however, professional advancement is limited, even though they may have excellent skills and knowledge in the field of nursing. In nursing education, registered practical nurses cannot use their education as the first step in the hierarchy, and continue on to become registered nurses. The two systems are not integrated in a manner that allows for easy up-skilling. In fact, as noted in an earlier discussion, nurse administrators hire unskilled individuals to work in areas of patient care. This double message—of higher education as a component of professionalism, and unskilled individuals can do some aspects of patient care—devalues a job that has been historically devalued through association with work that has been done in the home by women.

Nursing faculties in academic institutions provide socialisation through which education professionals control future nurses by imprinting on student nurses the ideal type. These faculties, in keeping with nursing leadership, see the BSN as the "true" professional nurse. By inferring that university-trained nurses are professional nurses whose practice is different from those trained in the college system, these faculty members have a platform where they can talk and write about the "professional nurse" or the

⤷ also for further discrimination.

106

"collegial nurse." It is their description of "this type of nurse" that nurse leaders and their peers in hospitals use as the behaviours expected of staff nurses. Nurses who wish to become part of the leadership in nursing may want to inculcate and cultivate the standards of these ideals in themselves in order to advance themselves. On the other hand, those individuals who are committed to working as a staff nurse, may choose not to follow the leadership or their values, since it does not meet their standards of what nursing work means.

There were two routes by which to enter nursing in Ontario, one through the college process, which results in a diploma, and the other through a four-year degree course acquired in a university. Hospital schools of nursing in Ontario were discontinued in 1973-74. The Moth's Nursing Task Force (1999) has, however, requested in 2005, that the CNO make the BSN the minimum baseline requirement for entry into the profession. This was achieved by students entering at the college level where they learn nursing skills, and then transferring to a university for other nursing knowledge.

There is linkage between colleges and universities in the educating of nurses. Since the vast majority of nurses are staff nurses, their buy-in to this aspect of professionalism is important, otherwise the conflict between these two groups will continue to influence the culture of nursing, and thus collegial behaviour. Conflict between the leadership and the staff nurse group can also increase cohesion among the staff nurse group, or alternately, promote hostile and stereotyping behaviours among staff nurses about their colleagues with degrees in nursing. The conflict is also responsible for degree nurses stereotyping diploma nurses, which has become a source of conflict among staff nurses.

As mentioned earlier, in the late 1970s, and again in the late 1990s, a shortage of staff nurses occurred in Toronto. During periods of nursing shortage, nurses are able to control their work hours, and are compensated with increased benefits. The tide turned in the late 1980s, and there was an abundance of staff nurses. At that time, nurses found themselves in a rapidly changing health care environment, and were sometimes downsized out of hospital employment, or were put into the 'casual' pool by nursing administration. With nurses in abundance, the power of the staff nurse within the hospital gave way in the face of the power of those in management, since their ability to select the preferred type of nurse for work in a hospital becomes greater in times of surplus.

While trying to hire new staff with degrees in nursing, the administration provided incentive packages for senior staff nurses to leave; these nurses were mostly non-BScN trained. This view was also voiced by the RNAO in their defence of the Hospital for Sick Children in Toronto when it terminated 17 experienced nurses, and hired younger nurses who had a BSN in their place (Toronto Star, July 9, 1998). This proved that connections existed among the elites within nursing. Since this hospital was not unionized, the ONA could not intervene on behalf of the nurses regarding union contracts, as they would have done in unionized hospitals.

In times of shortage of staff nurses, the rhetoric around the necessity for a professional nurse is reduced, and nursing management recruits nurses without degrees on account of need. The culture of the professional nurse who has a BScN takes a back seat to the need of having a staff nurse care for the sick within their institutions.

During the period of my survey, the issue of hiring university-educated nurses was central to the hiring decision discussions in nursing management, and therefore of parts of the construct of the culture of nursing within Ontario. By 1998, however, there was once again in Ontario a shortage of nurses, and again, staff nurses had more control over where they worked, and the number of hours worked. Staff nurses are encouraged to work overtime or have two jobs by choice, one full-time, and one working as a 'casual' nurse in another hospital. The CNO and ONA are aware of the practice but do not intervene as to the safety issues that accompany an overworked and exhausted staff. The structures of power within the profession and the hospital system turn a blind eye to this practice of overwork. It should also be noted that nurses who work at the bedside, and who are overworked due to staff shortages or workload, clearly have less time to be involved in developing themselves or their profession.

Feedback from staff nurses during interviews on the discussion around education systems meant hearing "the hands-on, versus the book-knowledge" arguments over and over again, even as late as 2004. On "Nurse net: A Global Forum for Nursing," the issue of whether a "nurse is a nurse", or a nurse is one who is credentialed, and more generally, the related issue of the "education of nurses," was discussed in forty-one e-mail communications. These discussions were similar to the discussions I encountered among staff nurses in Toronto. As a nurse who started as a diploma nurse from a hospital school of nursing, I felt that a nursing degree would not help me to develop the knowledge base that I needed in Mental

Health and Counselling. I looked at what would give me the best context for expanding and developing knowledge in psychiatry, and so chose a non-nursing degree.

From my own perspective as a diploma nurse, and as someone who had gone to university, both groups of nurses that I interviewed come from a specific world of training. My socialization having included both the hospital and university environments provided me with a comfort level in both worlds. Nurses in my sample made sarcastic remarks describing the "other" in terms of her or his status as a nurse. I found that non-degree nurses demeaned the skills of BScN nurses, who themselves demeaned diploma nurses as not understanding researched-based practice. This type of tension provides for a hostile, abusive work environment relating to an idealized vision of nursing, and stemming from a particular ideology around the work nurses should do.

The animosities that arose from these three types of education—hospital, college, and university—involved arguments based about stereotypes. Hospital-trained nurses believed that they had the most in-depth clinical background that allows them to fit easily into the workplace; and felt that the degree nurses have the academic credits but less skill at the bedside. Staff nurses from colleges with practical experience, also viewed those coming out of university to be weak at the bedside. On the other hand, BSN graduates tended to decry the fact that college and hospital graduates have difficulty in conceptualizing the holistic needs of patients; and that the latter are rewarded to not think but rather, to fit into the hospital mould.

This discourse about the definition of who is a professional nurse provides nursing with a hierarchical culture, with university-trained nurses at the top of the hierarchy. It also meant that experienced diploma nurses could be deprived of her/his ability to work, while a new graduate with a BSN would gain employment. This climate formed the basis of a large part of the acrimony that was aimed at the staff nurse. The statements below are in the words of nurses who addressed this issue via e-mail:

> Discussion about the "best" way to educate nurses probably started with Florence Nightingale when she suggested that nurses needed some type of systematic instruction. When I started in nursing, the BSN versus the diploma versus associate degree debate was raging. Now the issues seem to be related to graduate/specialty education, so perhaps the

profession is moving through a "normal" developmental process...I am finishing a doctoral degree, but not in nursing. This was a very considered decision after comparing curricula and trying to determine what education would best prepare me for what I wanted to do. I have a diploma in nursing, a bachelor and masters degree in nursing, and have practiced as a clinical specialist and taught clinical nursing in a baccalaureate program.... Legally, in the U.S., a nurse can still practice professional nursing with a diploma, an associate degree, or a bachelor degree (BSN). Perhaps that is the factor that continues to feed this controversy. Can you say that a BSN has the potential to contribute more to nursing than a diploma nurse with a bachelor degree in sociology? However, most graduate programs in nursing now require nursing degrees, so diverging from nursing before the doctoral level closes some doors. Within nursing, I think there is an attitude that the highest status is reserved for those with only nursing degrees. However, I remember a study reported in Nursing Outlook a few years ago that examined the research output of doctoral nurses and found that the type of doctoral degree was not significantly related to the amount of research activity. (D.B., August 1995)

I found the comments made on the Internet by D.B. similar to those made by nurses who have taken their degrees in other areas of higher learning. This includes comments that I too made in the past concerning the contributions we make to the profession of nursing.

In the past, nursing education in Ontario made it difficult to transfer credits from college courses to a nursing degree. Nurses from hospital schools or colleges had to start at the beginning and seats at the university were limited. Part-time studies are now available, and nurses have availed themselves of these programmes in order to upgrade to a BSN degree. Had the university made this available in the 1970s and 1980s, the issue of the BSN nurse would be less of a struggle. Today, nurses face the task of up-skilling credentials towards a graduate degree; this is compounded by the fact that spaces in graduate programs are limited. In addition, charges of racism have been levelled towards universities that do not have racialised nursing professors, and do not understand the need to have a diverse faculty.

Today in nursing, the contributions and the worth of the individual nurse are questioned by those within the profession, and by the nursing administration. Their scepticism is based, not purely on the grounds of how the nurse performs her/his work, but also on issues such as research, continuing education, and committee work. Most nurses who have worked for several years, and who do not have degrees often see experience as an important factor. They feel that these experiences give them status based on the holding of practical knowledge within the group at the unit level. New nurses to the unit ask them questions around care-giving issues, and these experienced nurses are sought out to orientate new staff nurses.

The following statement describes how nurses generally feel about the issue of nursing ability and experience:

> I have been a RN now for over 19 years and quite enjoy my job. To say that a 20-year-old BSN grad has more abilities then a 20-year veteran with the historical base of wisdom and a life-long learning in a multitude of interests makes for a less nurse than a BSN is simply wrong. I could clarify this post more so that it would not be easy to take cheap shots at, but I believe in whole that it has made my point and will leave it at that." (J., email communication)

Nurses are pitted against each other by administration when they advertise for staff. The comments below from the internet describe the annoyance and anger that are expressed within the profession for discrimination against advanced (diploma) nurses.

> In regards to your recent post I must add a few comments. The fighting between ADVANCED nurses and ones with less qualified education is an interesting one. (J., email communication)

> Apply for that position! You've already mentioned that it's illegal to say: "BSN required." So, make them prove that you don't qualify! And be very attuned to the possibility of a discrimination suit. (L., email communication)

These comments provide a picture of where nurses feel devalued.

111

This is the same type of behaviour that feminist researchers describe when exploring women's work—the devaluing of women because they did not meet the requirements of a patriarchal society. Requirements in nursing have changed over the years to reflect the same kinds of requirements that feminist research identified males using to define who is valued in the workplace.

Thirty years ago, it was the type of hospital, or the country in which the nurse was trained that made the difference in how s/he was assessed and valued as having the "right" skills. The assessment also depended on who was describing the incident or the skill-set.

During my training as a nurse, I have heard the need for nurses to unite. In hospital nursing schools, classmates become a surrogate family. At one time or another, we students comforted each other, complained amongst ourselves, and pulled each other out of tight spots. Perhaps bonding occurred within the group as students lived and worked together while training in hospitals. It is clear, however, that struggles within nursing have always existed in some form or another.

On the wards, now called units, students have experienced great power struggles and abuse when dealing with some of the senior staff nurses. Statements such as "You don't know," or "We do not do it this way" pointed out that we were less qualified or less experienced than those nurses who were senior to us. As students and as staff nurses, having our mistakes pointed out was a normal occurrence for us. The de-skilling and verbal abuse that occurs in nursing, would, if it occurred within a marriage be labelled as domestic violence — or the start of domestic violence, and would not be tolerated. In the nursing workplace, however, it is not viewed as violence when an individual's self esteem is violated.

My interviews with nurses let me know that this behaviour still existed and that in addition, judging and rating nurses based on their levels of education had become a major issue. Nurses with experience complained that they were passed over and new graduates were given choice positions. Another e-mail message states this division that I heard in my interviews:

> I think it is all of the above and more. BSN nurses seem better able to focus on nursing issues. AD and diploma seem more inclined to see nursing as physician assisting. Those, however are broad generalizations and don't include every-one. Some BSNs can't find their way out of a box and some

AAs or diploma nurses are very creative, nursing oriented practitioners. I think it has to do with the content of programs, the hospital orientation of the diploma and AA and the values modeled in the academic programs. (Barbara)

Staff nurses argue about education credentials only when the culture of the hospital values one type of staff over another. Most RNs would like to see this argument put to bed. The following e-mail is indicative of what I heard from many staff nurses during informal exchanges, indicating that bickering over status diminishes the power and divides the staff nurses as a group. Terry and L.S. state:

Let's stop the bickering and start working on credibility & respect for the profession as a whole. I have been an RN for five years and a CRNA for 15 years. It hasn't been too long ago that a nurse is a nurse was looked at as some big-breasted female who was "easy picking" for any doctor or anyone else for that matter that came along. The image has changed somewhat over the years. The nursing image will have to change dramatically in order to get the respect that it deserves. People change that! Our opinions do count and don't forget it. We have the power as a profession to be what we want to be. Keep it Up. (Terry, e-mail communication)

I really think that we need to examine our individual assumptions... and our profession's assumptions. There is much disquieting about our internal rancour, and it *does* ill become us to tear each other down.... But a) has bedside nursing become either a technical/vocation practice b) what might Nursing become if bedside care *were* to be relegated to a technical status... and the *professionals* cruised the units (much like physicians do now) and simply supervised, co-ordinated and developed the system of care; and' educated' the actual care-givers? (L.S.)

Nurses are not comfortable with the term "technical" nurse when they review the history of nursing:

> When we look at the "nurse," we see that as soon as her/his
> salary range goes up, those in power try to find another care-
> giver such as the LPN (licensed practical nurse). Now that
> the LPN wages have increased, those in power have once
> again created a title Personal Service Attendant (PSA) for a
> non-licensed individual to give care to patients. (D.L., A.V.,
> O.S, email communication)

The statements received via e-mail, globally speaking, are similar to
responses made in the interviews, focus groups and informal discussions
that I had with nurses in Toronto. In Ontario, diploma nurses are graduating year after year from community colleges, paid in part for their education by the Ontario taxpayers. As a health care resource, these nurses have
found it difficult (since 1990) to find employment—even as casual staff in
acute care institutions—when cutbacks occurred in hospitals within Metro
Toronto. Many left the province to work in other areas of North America.
The question of why the government of Ontario continues to fund these
programmes at the college level was not being addressed until 1999 (RNAO
1999). In times of scarcity, however, these same hospitals are eager to hire
diploma-educated nurses. Once again in 1998, because of a nursing shortage, diploma nurses were hired by hospitals in Toronto.

    Actions within the profession that produce the ideal nurse based on
higher education promote discrimination, exclusion, and differentiation.
This environment will not promote collegial behaviour but instead, creates
a toxic work environment. As several feminist noted in the 1960s, patriarchal discourses on work devalued women's work (see Jacobs 2002). Today
we find that within a female dominated profession the discourse has not
changed in terms of valuing work, and encouraging practices that heighten
women's shared consciousness.

Norms and Values Around Relationships and Promotions

Within the culture of nursing, there is a correlation between white privilege,
curricula (Hagey and MacKay 2000) and promotions. In the hierarchical
scheme of nursing, where whiteness is at the top, nurses who are further
from the centre of power—mostly those from racialised communities—are
excluded from resources. Those in power can use their positions to target
minority nurses, while looking the other way on behalf of nurses whom

they wish to mentor, and who identify with the dominant group. Perhaps the most important observation is that nursing programs for higher education do not necessarily serve to reduce racism, or class inequality but instead, serve to maintain the status quo. Staff nurses who are loyal to leaders within the hospital are oriented to the positions of power, allowing them to learn leadership roles, and are given the opportunity to manage others. Although authority relations are, on paper, based on rational standards and rules, and have an impersonal character, in practice, nurse leaders use privilege in decision-making.

For the majority of staff nurses, rules and standards impose discipline and control, and leave little room for discretion and individual initiative. A closer look reveals, however, that these standards and rules as applied by those who are in change of staff nurses demonstrate discretion and privilege. An example of how those in authority exercise considerable discretion and discrimination is described by one interviewee as occurring "…when a qualified experienced racialised nurse who requested to work as an interim manager is bypassed and nursing management appoints a less experienced white nurse for the position" (OS).

Based on years of observation, participation, and interviews for this research, I have found that informal circles of communication and interaction by those who hold positions of power within nursing are like the classic "old boys network." This network excludes many staff nurses, as well as minorities in management from significant information that flows through these networks. Those in power and those close to them exchange information about data, services, job prospects, and advancement possibilities. Staff nurses' access to these networks is limited, leaving them to rely on formal communication, such as announcements and memos. Informal gossip or information may never appear in public for all nurses; or it may come too late for other than the chosen group to apply for positions. Since information is power, those who control information are power brokers. At all levels of the profession, the manager determines relationships between the manager and the managed. Mentorship is one way of developing new leaders, and racialised nurses point to how senior white managers mentor specific white staff nurses who are part of the dominant group.

The complaints system is a factor for all nurses in their professional lives. Since this system has the potential to affect the livelihood of an individual nurse involved within it, the very fact of knowing of its existence and how it works, was, and is, experienced as coercive. Nurses at the management level, however, are seldom threatened with the targets of complaints as they rarely provide patient care; it is the nurse manager who receive complaints of alleged staff misconduct, and they are the ones who repor staff to the CNO.

In a landmark Human Rights Case in May 1994 agains Northwestern General Hospital in Toronto (Das Gupta 1996; Cooks 2000 racialised nurses stated that there were more complaints against them thar against their white counterparts. The affects of racism have not been wel documented, in terms of cost to the health care system, and so the ful impact of the over-reporting of racialised nurses is yet to be determined.

Procedures and policies are in place in every hospital, yet the affect: of racism are not documented. Some hospitals have diversity managers whc speak of feeling unsupported in their positions, and report receiving 'hate mail' for investigating human rights violations within the hospital. An envi ronment, in which basic rights are viewed as negative according to 'hate mail' received, is indicative of a toxic workplace. Documenting the affect: of racism would make for positive changes in the workplace, for justice i: recognizing the realities of racism and oppression. Injustice is structured institutionalized, and systemic.

At other times, patients, their families, or a visitor can report a nurse to the CNO. The formal complaints to the CNO can be expensive for the staff nurse if she/he retains a lawyer to defend against the allegation. Unlike a patient's civil law suit, wherein the hospital provides legal counsel, the nurse is on her own when a complaint is lodged against her or him at the CNO, unless she/he is a member of the RNAO or the ONA. For example the college charged a nurse, (J.M.) for "yelling at a patient." Although thi: was not true, the process necessitated a lawyer who was paid by the RNAO The physician in charge, the manager, and several peers supported the nurse in writing. The investigation lasted six months, with the CNO interviewing the physician and the nurse's peers. Although found not guilty, the CNC stated that the nurse should not have spoken to the patient. The RNAO paic out $2,500.00 for the nurse's defence and the lawyer informed the nurse tc drop the issue, as "the CNO has to listen to the public so they would state that." Not unexpectedly, the nurse reported feeling stressed over the ordeal

This legal aspect of nursing brings to the profession a culture o: legalism. Within this culture, elements of social control also exist, and car be traced to the policy actions taken by agents of the structures that make up the profession. In many cases, staff nurses are well aware of the constraints that are part of nursing culture; and in order to work within the standards and policies, will adapt some of their own values to fit these constraints. Discipline is assured by a set of rules that are intended to adjust the staff nurse's behaviour, and often, this implies a use of power. It is a situation whereby nurse leaders have power as they set policy, and as they interact through their network. Given the structural organization of nursing, and on account of the sheer number of the rank and file staff nurses, direct democratic participation is technically impossible. I have observed only a small group of staff nurses who involve themselves in the professional structure, while the majority stay silent and feel alienated.

Professional standards are also a form of social control within nursing as they can be used to obstruct, or harass ethnic and racial minority nurses, or nurses who fall into disfavour with those in management positions. Minority nurses (C.J., S.K., N.S.) reported how management made complaints to the CNO regarding their patient care, resulting in expensive legal fees as they defended themselves. These nurses were distressed that when the cases were dropped, those in management did not suffer any consequences on account of their allegations. They felt targeted because they had stood up to their managers, and as a result, standards of behaviour were used to harass them.

Standards of behaviour can also be used to promote an individual by viewing their behaviour in such a way that it lines up with professional standards. In fact, it was sometimes evident in my everyday life as a nurse, that any negative behaviour by those who were chosen for promotion was overlooked. Even though open contests (that is, postings) may exist as part of public and organizational standards, it is common to sponsor like-minded, and culturally/racially similar professional nurses to advance within the system. This is an example of how elites recruit and keep under close supervision those who can be thoroughly indoctrinated in the culture and who can then thereby become part of their group (Turner 1977).

It is only on paper that the concept of "open" competition appears as the system of advancement. In practice, the sponsorship system is how one is actually promoted. It is more usual that when nurses achieve a higher position in the organization, it is because of whom they know and not what they know. Clearly, mobility-oriented staff nurses, and many educated minority nurses who have not been incorporated into higher-level cliques, often do not win positions in open competition. The following account shows the experience of being incorporated and developed by a supervisor in nursing, as one chosen to take on a leadership role:

> My day-to-day activities were a process of developing my skills. Conferences, extra training, and other experiences that could develop me were provided at no cost to me. My mentor in psychiatry gave me opportunities to lead as a charge nurse and made sure that he taught me the role of a charge nurse. I grew and became a nurse manager and was given opportunities.

When new management arrived and racialised nurse managers were targeted:

> I was considered the outsider and experienced targeting and exclusion. My staff was called into the senior nursing administration and asked to share their views about how I ran the unit. All staff related incidents were related to my lack of judgement. When I checked with other managers, this behaviour did not extend to them. In fact, peer managers would document on me, while any problems I had regarding issues or behaviours would be discounted and told to deal with them directly. Conference time was provided but limited compared to the other managers. Information was withheld and when change occurred within the nursing program it was not provided at the same time as the other managers. I was being set-up for failure (J.M. 1997)

The sponsorship system is an underground network in which those chosen by elites within nursing may be freed from the strain of competitive struggles all the while, her or his deficiencies are covered up in order that this individual, whom they have taken into the inner circle, can appear to others as one with professional qualities. This is a structured, institutionalized, and systemic manner in which white privilege works, and how racism and injustice deny 'the other' the same opportunities as their white counterparts.

The following are two examples given by staff nurses that describe how they saw their experiences, and provides more insight into sponsorship within nursing:

D.P. without experience as an educator was chosen over several evening coordinators to become an educator in psychiatry, even though all her experience were in cardiac critical care. With less education and experience in psychiatry her mistakes were covered up. When complaints were voiced about her abilities, they were not dealt with. There was no recourse. She was the expert in the area of psychiatry without having the skills and knowledge. I had more experience and knowledge in psychiatry and yet she was worked into the position without the position posted. (B.D., staff nurse psychiatry, 1996)

S.J., a two-year diploma nurse with a BA in Psychology and an MBA, was given a Director of Nursing position within our hospital. She displaced another Director who was told that she was too old to change. S.J. did not have any management experience and was brought in by her friend, a new V-P. S.J. worked as a work load measurement consultant before she arrived at our hospital. Nurses within the hospital were expected to upgrade their education to a BSN level and nurse managers were targeted if they did not have a BSN. But this woman, and those who were part of the group around the Senior Nursing Administration, they got away with a different educational level and were given positions even when they did not have the same level of experience. They got a lot of perks. (P.M., staff nurse, cardiac care, 1996)

As in any sponsored situation, these nurses do compete in an "open" competition, knowing they have an edge over those who lack the backing of the leadership. In order to hire them, the sponsors can change the focus of their criteria in order to get their nurse hired. This assertion is embedded in statements provided by another staff nurse, who is a minority nurse. B.J. stated:

I went for the interview for a management position within the hospital. I had more education, experience, and the qualification for the position on paper. The committee chosen to

119

interview the others and myself for the position were hand picked and the interviewers knew the questions. The Director of Nursing in charge of this process called the chosen individual prior to the interview and went over the questions with the individual. The nurse leaders on the committee all provided this individual with extra points over me, while the other members of the committee such as physicians gave me points that put me in the lead. In the end, the individual won with a couple of points over me. The contest was unfair but there was nothing I could do. On paper they made it look fair. They know whom they want in positions and contain those of us in staff nurse positions with little access to these positions. They try to treat you as if you do not have a brain. (B.J., 1995)

To stop open dissent among the majority of nurses, nursing leaders present a system whereby seemingly objective open contests exist, with a point system for ranking applicants. B.J. was able to challenge the decision concerning her application, only to find out that the procedure "was objective," and there was nothing that could be done. Among the strong "grapevine" that exists in most Toronto hospitals, it is said that there are leaks from hiring committees concerning unfairness, and preparing staff for positions, while harassing others. The grapevine suggests that the behaviour described by B.J., (that a nursing leader chose the individual that she wanted, and that there was a system of "unprofessional actions" to achieve the desired results) is indicative of a wider pattern.

The argument proposed here is that the nursing profession in Ontario was, and remains at a level whereby identification with the leadership and their ideal type is important because of the norm of sponsored mobility that exists among the leadership. Leadership behaviour provides a much clearer picture of a closed professional culture in which like-minded individuals promote their own kind. This process was and is also used to exclude minorities, both at the educational level of nursing, and within the management level of the profession. That is why "the Cappuccino Principle"—white on top, brown on the bottom—speaks to how this profession continues to be divided along racialised lines. The suppression of minority nurses, the lack of minority nurses in positions of power in every structure of nursing, can only be viewed as racism.

The Value of the Real Nurse:
Who is a Real Nurse? A View from the Staff Nurses

Staff nurses state that the hiring of educators, planners, and other non-bedside nurses is a misuse of government funds within hospitals. The educators, managers, and clinical specialist often have graduate degrees in nursing. Increasing in number during cutbacks of bedside nurses, these nurses are resented by nurses working at the bedside. In many discussions, staff nurses viewed the tasks that are outside the caring of patients as less valuable and "more frills." Many staff nurses agree with the statement that nurse leaders "come through the units/wards like doctors." The following are comments regarding non-bedside nurses:

> I don't know what she does on this unit. She is supposed to be with the staff but she is seeing patients, and acting like another manager. (E.S., staff nurse, 1997)

> The Clinical Nursing Educator that we have is trying to make us look like we do not know what we are doing and tries to train us in procedures that we know. They try to make work for themselves at our expense. (D.O., staff nurse, 1996)

> The nurse in infectious control tries to act like she is above us. When we have a problem she wants paper work but does not come up to problem solve with us. (M.P., staff nurse, 1996)

Rather than viewing these nurses as part of a team, staff nurses find them in the way of their work, and do not think that they represent the best use of scarce financial resources:

> I find them making work for themselves. The clinical resource does not ask what we want to learn. She put on a subject that we already knew and only two staff went to her lecture. They want to give us a certificate if we attend which is not worth anything. (E.S., staff nurse, 1997)

> I was so mad with the educator. She is jealous of my role as a team leader. I went in and asked her what her problem was

and told her that what I did was for my patients. She tried to be sweet and look like she did not know what was the problem. I told her that she did not answer her pager and that she was not around when the staff needed her. She is such a pain.... (O.S., staff nurse, 1997)

The conflicts about why staff nurses need educators and how they view them is important. When nurses view their work as distant from their view of patient care and more a part of administration, once again other staff nurses discounts this nurse as having any value. In their discussions, staff nurses stated that they did not feel helped by clinical educators or by nurses who worked in areas such as risk management, quality programmes, and development of nursing practice.

Staff nurses voiced distrust and did not want to have close interactions with these nurses. These interactions as reported by staff nurses were described at times to be hostile or else distant. Nurse Unit Mangers or Nursing Managers fared better, as they interact with staff nurses around direct patient care issues. Therefore, the value of helping each other is part of their culture.

The interviewees were asked the question in the survey: "Do nurses help each other when problems occur?" Those staff nurses' who responded positively expressed the view that nurses help each other out, showing that the positive value of "helping out" is high. The results were: when problems arise, 20% "always" help each other, and 51.5% "often" help each other. Perhaps the reason that staff nurses do not extend this attitude to clinical education, or to other areas as described, is arguably traceable to the tension that exists between staff nurses and the professional elite.

Those staff nurses who have trained in colleges or at hospitals have stated that they find themselves looked down upon by the nurses in positions of power (such as managers, consultants, and clinical educators) who come into patient care areas looking at issues, not as co-equals but as "know-it-all" experts. The bickering becomes more acute when employees fear for their future within the institution, and feel monitored by these nurses. The result of the twin elements of powerlessness and fear is infighting at the unit level, and within the institution. This culminates in an aspect of nursing culture wherein conflict appears to exist at the hospital level but has its roots in academia; it is also rooted in the prejudice held by staff nurses toward those who come from universities and are not believed to be a part of the provision of direct patient care.

The Cultural Value of Autonomy

As with other professions, nursing has developed a view of itself. Changing the image from a semi-professional to a more professional one has been an absorbing factor for nurses who are located further up the hierarchy. As stated earlier, nurses in the CNO, the RNAO, and those working, either as educators at universities, or in administrative positions, are those with decision-making power within the profession. Many participants in this research view the leadership as elites within the profession and do not interact with them. These nurse leaders are also the individuals who speak out for nursing autonomy. The CNO and the RNAO both argue for autonomy through professionalism.

As a member of the occupation, the issues of back-stage behaviour provided me with a view that makes this writer see it differently from those who merely know of it through hearsay. Perhaps we have within the profession, both semi-professional and professional nurses. Through the CNO, the nurse has control over her/his own fate, and the occupation has built a body of professional knowledge that fulfils the criteria for professionalisation put forward as to who counts as a professional (see, e.g., Hughes et al., 1958).

The work of the staff nurse is complex, scientific, caring, and demanding. Unlike physicians, however, nurses at the bedside are still undervalued. They do not have autonomy, as despite the proliferation in theoretical and technical knowledge within the profession, they must follow the doctor's orders (Grow 1991; Armstrong and Armstrong 1996). Therefore, staff nurses at the bedside can also be viewed as semi-professional due to the lack of autonomy over their work.

It can also be argued that the major portions of nursing accomplishment have been built on the backs of the staff nurses. Staff nurses and student nurses are also participants in research, the credit for which goes to the nurse researchers. As pointed out by several nurses, research-based practice within hospitals usually comes from the top down, as pointed out by several nurses:

> They take an idea that comes from an Ivory Tower, bring it to our unit or want to change a system, and then we have to fill the forms. She comes and collects the forms and two to four of them in management get together write it, up get it

123

published with no credit to us nurses who had to do the work, had to learn the new system.... (V.D., interview, 1995)

When they changed our staffing patterns with unskilled workers they made us fill out forms on all our shifts. With the new unskilled workers we had more work and yet we had to do this. Guess what happened? They used the stuff that we got, and published it to promote themselves. They bring in other researchers and let them use us to get research when we have so much to do and are so busy.... (D.C., interview, 1996)

V.D. and D.C. stated in the interview what I heard many staff nurses discuss about research within their work hours. To speak out against it openly is problematic for the nurse. The reality is, however, that the outcome of the research has no impact on their success. When I asked some individuals why they were participating in my research, the responses I received were: "I am choosing to speak to you," "I like what you are doing," "it is my issue too," and "you talk to me on my time." I also heard from staff nurses that nurse leaders used hospital time to advance themselves by publishing, while they were short staffed, overworked, and not part of the small group who got their names on "the paper." Many of the staff nurses were part-time students and needed the same exposure to academic life as those in management. Instead, they complain that they are used to collect data, which is then used by management for their projects.

The hierarchy of nursing within hospitals has been slow to follow decentralization when it comes to the decision-making at the staff nurse level. This type of decision-making is conducive to the full use of their expertise, knowledge, and skills. Autonomy as part of nursing culture is only relevant when all nurses are equal in worth, rather than as currently whereby the elite class seeks autonomy for the profession in order to acquire more power for themselves.

In the next section I will deal with the construction of the culture of the staff nurses' work environment and their feelings around this issue. When we examine the professional culture, we see a culture based on rules, formal in communication and organized in a bureaucratic hierarchy. In viewing the value of autonomy, the hospital community has an effect on the culture of nursing.

124

Constructing the Hospital Community: The Affect on Nursing Culture

Over the last fifteen years, news reports regarding the crisis in health care in Ontario have been commonplace. The policies of the federal and provincial governments, originating with the cutbacks in transfer payments from the federal government to the provinces in general, have provided for unstable funding. In Ontario, however, despite the cutbacks to hospitals, the funding in health has increased each year. In 1999, the MoH provided $325 million earmarked for nursing (RNAO 1999, 12). The RNAO used public advocacy and the insufficient amount of nursing care (RNAO 1999, 2) and found that the public blamed the government as being primarily responsible for the situation; the public also levelled blame at health-care administrators and their "bottom-line cost-reduction approach" (1999, 2). Downsizing and restructuring, as well as internal budget cutting that hospitals have been undergoing since the early 1990s have brought uncertainty and stressors to those working in acute care sectors; this is especially so for nurses who work directly with patients. This workplace environment has an affect on nursing culture at the staff nurse level, as informal organizations based on friendship groups and interactions are disrupted through downsizing and restructuring.

Acute Care Hospitals

Hospitals have become corporate entities. The expansion of the utilization of technological devices in medicine and of information systems in the hospital system has resulted in the rethinking of resource allocation in a context in which professionals work together for patient care. In the document *The Future of Health Care* (2001) the Hospitals of Ontario stated that they serve approximately 1.2 million inpatients and care for 13.5 million outpatients. The types of hospitals include teaching and specialty hospitals, small hospitals, community hospitals, mental health hospitals, rehabilitation hospitals, and chronic care hospitals. For the most part, the provincial and federal governments fund health care in Canada, with more than 70% of a hospital's budget going to the salaries and benefits of the people who work there. The largest departments in any hospital are those of Patient Services, which in the past were known as Nursing Divisions. Thus, the bulk of a hospital's budget goes to the operation of nursing care. With the progress of science and technology, there is competition with the paradigm of "hands-on" care. Coupled with this is the fact that a technological revolution of medical devices has taken place within a culture of rationalisation; and this has resulted in an attack on the fundamentals of the traditional paradigm of a holistic approach to healthcare.

Professional and non-professional staff, such as those working in housekeeping, laundry, and so forth delivers the healthcare within a hospital. Those who provide services include radiology/medical imaging, laboratories, physiotherapy, social work, pharmacy, and dieticians. The size of the departments and their ability to influence what happens within each hospital varies. I have heard other departments expressing views of the nursing departments as having power, due to the fact that most of the budget is allocated to the nursing division. Although they are not employees of the hospital, through written orders, the organized medical profession uses the hospital budget for the care of their patients. Most medical care given to patients by physicians comes out of government revenues, through the Ontario Health Insurance Plan (OHIP) or a hospital budget. In a funding crisis, professional self-interest motivates health care professionals in their decisions on how the "funding pie" gets cut. Administrators must balance the needs of the sick, the community, the interests of each group, and their own interests, within the priorities of the government of the day.

In the *Future of Health Care*, one of the principles of care discussed is that professionals work together. The document states:

> Health care providers from all aspects of health care must work together to find the best and most cost effective means of treating patients in their communities. This includes providing support to the front-line professionals who make health care what it is today. (Government of Canada 2001)

The vision of the Hospitals of Ontario is as an environment in which front-line professionals are supported and valued. Nurses are experiencing conflicted feelings regarding the message that is written when they find themselves in an environment in which they lack role autonomy, and where they experience racism and abuse. Team work, team approach, and working together for the patient are some of the ideals that managers and executives use for bringing all those employed for the patient together on equal footing. Within the team, however, the staff nurse does not feel respected, as team members look to nurses in management for answers, rather than to the staff nurse.

Relationships between individuals in the organization differ because of overt inequality in power. Current political strategies for empowering the staff nurse include forming coalitions with certain physicians who admit patients to their unit. In order for the staff nurse to gain power within the health care team, bargaining and lobbying with the physicians become a part of the norms governing nurse-physician relationships.

Hospital environments are complex organizations with differentiation of tasks assigned to occupational groups with formal roles. At times, these groups come together as a team, with patient care as their main focus; and at other times they divide the institution into distinctive groups. There are physicians, nurses, dietary staff, physiotherapists, social workers, discharge planners, speech therapists, lab technicians, medical imagining staff, housekeeping staff, and clerical staff, to name a few. With an increase in power, there is a pressure to change their roles or the tasks they do. As a staff nurse, I found that the nurses in speciality areas, such as psychiatry, emergency, and critical care, had more input into the treatment and discussion around patient care than did those nurses working on the medical and surgical units; they were often not heard by the physicians. Many of these physicians had egos that could not handle a nurse acting without his or her direct orders. This was especially so if the nurse proved to have knowledge or competence that the physician did not have, or neglected to apply in the situation. Given the fact that medicine and nursing are bound by function, some doctor-nurse combinations act as a team. Physicians that welcome and encourage nurses to do what was best for "their" patient provided a team approach to patient care.

There are physicians who like to give orders to nurses concerning the care of patients; these come in a formalized ritual, such as "order forms". In this case, the physician writes an order that nurses are expected to carry out "in the best interest" of patient care. Historically, physicians have been the primary power bases in any hospital, and so taking their cue from physicians other professionals within the hospital will make demands on the staff nurse. I have heard other professionals say to a staff nurse, "Put this report in Mr. X's chart," when they could have done this themselves. A nurse who graduated in 1956 made this statement on the collegial survey:

> My family did not encourage me to become a nurse, I
> became a nurse cause I enjoyed looking after people. The

best thing about being a nurse is to have continuous learning progress with progression in the profession. One thing I dislike about nursing is being talked down to by patients and physicians and those professions that fly through the unit. (No.11 survey)

The physician is always the "doctor in charge" of the "case", but must work within the team around the delivery of patient-care. Patient-care teams exist in many hospitals, and are part of the accreditation of a hospital. The barriers that limit interaction and the real development of a team approach within most hospitals should be considered as "turf wars". A major reason is the inability to have open communication without the fear of dysfunctional consequences on the part of one or more team members. Senior management often cites teamwork in order to promote a culture of co-operation, and patient-centred care. Hospital administrators want patient-care teams to function in order that they adhere to standards of accreditation. Those working within the team have expectations, however, that their role within the team will not be targeted when a crisis occurs.

The patterns of interactions are still hierarchical, allowing both physicians and management to have the upper hand over the staff nurse within these teams.

Each institution has a history and culture that renders it distinctive in terms of how patient care is delivered. With downsizing in 1997 in Ontario, there is a general culture of displacement, and disruptions, plus increased workloads for the staff. Relationships within such a workplace are not the kind where inter-professional relationships can be collaborative and supportive. With a long history of rivalry for power among the different professional groups, this new development makes for a far more hostile and competitive environment for the team members within a department. Again, the organizational structure of the hospital is one that fosters vertical interaction, and reduces communication between the various groups. All staff members were aware that their future was uncertain, and this tension within departments made it difficult to work together to put patients first.

Department heads, or unit managers, are located in the organizational chart in such a way that allows for what I call an "upward communication pattern," in which a message is conveyed to the one unit, and then down to the worker. As a culture of problem solving, this communicative pattern prevents interactions with other individuals without the knowledge of the manager of the unit that first receives the message.

Union agreements also play a part in how issues are resolved, and affect the culture of problem solving, because staff nurses had a process that had to go beyond the unit, and involved Human Resources Departments. Some staff nurses felt that the union did not represent their interests, and in fact acted much like management. Since each party has to involve management, the manner in which unit specific problems are solved can at times promote an environment that is contrary to direct peer communication. The notion of empowering nurses to communicate and deal with issues produces a complex problem when the resolution process is taken away from them. Staff nurses still have to interpret which problem invokes the different problem solving processes, and can be disciplined if she or he does not use the right process.

To understand how decisions are made in each hospital requires a map of the organizational decision-making process and rules, and an indication of the agents who guide this process. There are the hospital-wide committees, board committees, department committees, and unit committees. For the staff nurse, learning and implementing this work takes time from their patient care.

Policy is usually made in a committee within the hospital but in reality, the structure of decision-making is unclear. On paper, however, it is fairly easy to outline decision-making structures. Informal meetings in the background do make strategies and alliances for what takes place formally. Staff nurses do not know what is decided by these committees until after the fact, and management has been known to not admit that they do not always make the best decisions—that is, not wanting to admit that the outcomes could have been achieved in another way with more input from stake holders—and that once those in power make a decision about an issue it is a "done deal." Validation then takes place as to why management's decision is a good decision. B.H., a staff nurse, related her view on policy making:

> A policy was made around signing off narcotics at the staff nurse level, a rather punitive policy, which was the brainchild of the Director of Nursing Practice (DON). Unit Nursing Managers then became part of the decision. The letters to the staff were designed by the DON. The managers gave the staff the letters even if they had signed off the sheet but forgot to put the doctor's name, a minor issue. The drug count was in order, but if there was a little error, the staff

nurse was to receive a letter. On the fourth occurrence the staff would loose his/her job. The staff nurses fought to have this changed with little results. The Director of Human Resources was approached, with no success. Staff nurses argued that there were no errors but [rather] documentation issues. That these letters made them look like they were misusing drugs and misleading. Support was given to management and not the staff. When the managers found the staff angry, and upset at them, they bent the policy without informing the DON. Some managers called the staff in to finish the documentation. In the end, because it suited the Nurse Managers, they requested a policy change after the DON had left the employ of the hospital. (V.D., interview, 1996)

A type of decision-making style with an inability to correct wrong decisions creates a culture of distrust and anger for staff nurses. In many decision-making committees, physicians still have input through the Medical Advisory Committee in all Ontario hospitals. In the 1990s, employee participation increased both by law and through Hospital Accreditation Standards. Hospital Accreditation made it the goal and objective to put patients first and at the centre of all decisions. Accreditation has resulted in the bringing in of more input from the staff nurse in these accreditation teams. There are usually, however, more professionals from other disciplines, and more managers than staff nurses. When staff nurses do not attend, it leaves nursing management as the only spokesperson for nursing, and once again allows them to take the lead in decision-making. In the team that I observed, staff nurses with their shift work and bedside care found it hard to attend meetings, while management and other employees could take the time to attend them.

The factor of "time versus tasks" plays an important role for the staff nurse when it comes to making a choice between committee meetings and patient care. When given the chance, staff nurses have a lot to offer: they voice their impressions, opinions, and concerns when they do attend meetings, adding a great deal to the discussion at hand. Given their level on the hierarchical ladder, however, management at meetings need to be sensitive and aware of their tone and actions, in order to provide a culture that is safe for the staff nurse to contribute.

At one general meeting, for example, I witnessed a senior nursing administrator admonish a staff nurse in public for not opening her eyes while this administrator was talking. It was a 'dressing down' that brought attention to the individual in public, who, it turned out, was closing her eyes due to eye strain. The staff nurse remained silent and thereafter participated less in public meetings. Such public, personally negative comments in committees or general meetings tend to make those in power have control over the agenda, as well as the outcomes.

I have also seen situations where nursing leaders have brought staff into committees as equal participants, and encouraged them to voice their ideas and knowledge. When this occurs, staff nurses enjoy their contribution to committee work and have informed me of this during my conversations with them at lunch meetings. Many of these leaders have acted as role models, and have provided an open environment that allows for different views. This makes for a collegial culture wherein conflictual ideas are viewed as a part of a positive process.

positive point (at last!)

Staff nurses have stated, however, that the hospital hierarchy, with its layers of power and accountability, resulted in them not wanting to "rock the boat," and so for various reasons, they usually did not challenge those in power at the committee level. The following was what a staff nurse stated when asked about committee work:

> There are so many committees in our hospital. Some nurses like going to committees but are not on the unit to do their work and they do not replace them. I have been to a committee on quality management that worked because we all had something to say and the leader was good. She let everyone have their say. But when you go to a committee where the V-P or Director is the leader you cannot really say how you feel because they come with an agenda and want you to agree to what they have to say. They say they want feedback but only to a certain degree…Especially if they want to change something, or change a policy. Usually there are a lot more management staff and a few of us staff nurses in the committee. The committee structure is a way of trying to get staff feedback but it is difficult. When you go back to the unit, your co-workers are upset with the policy or what happened at the committee. I feel that I have let them down. (M.K., medical nurse, 1995)

Nevertheless, some hospitals have shared governance where input from staff nurses is desired. The history of distrust has resulted in staff nurses not taking this as a new beginning, and hence, do not attempt to change the culture of the organization through participation. As D.O. (staff nurse surgical, 1997) and P.M. (staff nurse medical, 1997) informed me, they did not believe or trust administration, nor did they think they could change outcomes. Low morale among staff nurses and a heavy workload contributed to a feeling of powerlessness in which they view their work world as one where their opinions did not count. Another staff nurse, when asked about committee work, stated:

> What is the use for us to give our feedback and our concerns at meetings, and they do what they want to do in the end. Management sets the agenda.... These meetings, when we go back, our work is still there while managers and other people like the social worker and pharmacy can do it the next day. I can't be bothered with their meetings any more (O.S., surgical nurse, 1995)

Committee work is two-sided: it helps staff nurses advance and become known to management, while it also overworks the nurse involved. Management, on the other hand, was allocated time for meetings, while the staff nurse still had to return to the patient who needed treatment and care and whom she/he had left behind. Many staff nurses felt a sense of guilt if they had long spells away from their patients. Thus, although committees are an opening for staff nurses to participate in discussions, they can only make use of the opportunity if their workload is reduced.

In hospitals, the front-line professionals are the staff nurses. In "End of the Nurse," an essay in the *Registered Nurse*, a staff nurse describes the atmosphere experienced while at work. She states:

> My mother is a nurse. So were her mother and grandmother. At one time following the family tradition, I had similar ambitions. These aspirations of mine were, however, adamantly discouraged by my mother. It might appear as though my mother dislikes her profession, but that is not the case. She loves nursing and is very good at it. She merely feels that the nursing profession does not receive the recog-

nition it deserves from the rest of the health care community. (April-May 1992, 13)

This feeling of not receiving recognition was also voiced in my interviews and group discussions. When discussing work over coffee, a staff nurse told me that:

> ...the hospital is like a pan of cookie dough. All these other professionals cut their cookies out [what they want to do for patients] and leave us the edges. They come to work Monday to Friday from eight a.m. 'till five p.m. and when they leave their cookies [work], we take care of them. When they return on Monday, they like to tell us what we are not doing or what to do for that patient.

The patient is taken care of by the staff nurse, twenty-four hours a day, yet they feel that other hospital workers, who come on the units during business hours, treat them "as if we do not have a brain in our heads." During the evenings, throughout the night, and on weekends, the nurses are in charge of their units; it is their feeling, however, that those who only work "office hours" do not respect them for the amount of this responsibility.

This environment also produces an organizational culture wherein staff nurses find themselves finishing or checking to see if other professionals have completed tasks. The lack of perceived recognition for their role results in an "us and them" mentality—as well as in some women leaving nursing.

The hospital environment is based on power, status, and prestige, all of which are sometimes unrelated to the organizational goals. The lack of attention by senior administration to the staff nurse group, and administrators allowing nursing management to speak for this group in committees, has helped create a hierarchical culture in which the staff nurse feels powerless.

The Nature of Abuse and the Culture that Supports These Actions

Nursing is about caring, and so it is perhaps not surprising that the nature of abuse, and the culture that supports abusive behaviour are seldom discussed. Nurses do, however, experience abuse, and know it to be a part of the culture. They describe as coming from different individuals, and in different forms. Many nurses recalled at least one incident during formal interviews, or in discussion groups. The abuse with which nurses come in contact originates primarily from physicians, patients, and patients' families. Some staff nurses recalled that some of their peers have also been abusive to them.

The CNO has a programme whose theme is "Speak Out to Stop Abuse." The programme emerged as a result of CNO research that showed that when a nurse intervenes during an incident of client abuse, the abuse stops. Thus, the programme is intended to empower nurses, to get them involved, and to protect their clients, their colleagues, and themselves. This programme focuses on helping nurses to recognize warning signs, and on their obligation to speak out about abuse by others. For this organization, abuse can be emotional, verbal, physical and sexual. Racism, however, is not formulated as abuse (CNO web page, 2004).

When racism is not viewed as part of abuse by the College, then it is regulated to a space on its own. Racism then has its own identity, and is not part of "Speak Out to Stop Abuse." Perhaps this is because the CNO is made up of individuals of the dominant group, and the experience of abuse, and the experience of racism are not one and the same for them. For racialised individuals, racism is trauma, just like any other abuse. Once again, this is part of "the Cappuccino Principle"—white on top, brown on the bottom, which provides a different context to racist behaviour, and the naming of it.

Physicians are often a source of abuse for staff nurses. Apart from yelling and threatening staff nurses that they will report them, staff nurses state that they feel harassed and pushed by physicians. As one staff nurse reported, "You have more rights on the street than in a hospital." Nurses report that they find the workplace to be unsafe, with a lack of follow-up. Hospitals, they say, are slow to act on their behalf; and I have seen this first hand, when nurses have wanted to file a complaint. They usually do not find support from hospital administrators, who tend to make excuses for the unacceptable behaviour. This response from management in turn creates low staff morale.

A nurse recounted that a physician, when requested to sign his orders, threw the chart at her and walked away. Although this incident was reported, the outcome was one of silence from management. Staff nurses reported that the lack of intervention by management when physicians

134

yelled and/or threatened them made their "jobs a lot harder, and a source of irritation." Physicians have more power than nurses within the hospital, and management's actions reinforce their sense of powerlessness.

Another source of abuse comes from patients and visitors—anger from patients towards the nursing staff when they do not get their needs met; or yelling on the part of family members who are concerned about the care provided—have been related to me by staff nurses as demonstrations of verbal abuse. Patients can also complain about their actions to the nurse manager, administration, the social worker, the physician, or anyone with whom the patient comes in contact during their hospital stay. As a result, the nurse is the individual questioned: "Why... have you not done this?" in most instances.

Although hospitals state that they are cutting costs and not quality, patients expect the same attention from the nurse at the bedside. As stated by a nurse:

> Call bells cannot be answered when we are busy with another patient. The family gets angry at us and thinks we are sitting and doing nothing. We rush from one patient to another giving medication. We are the ones who the patient and the patient's family complain about to and do not know how may staff cutbacks have taken place. The manager always takes the patient's concern because they are concerned about risk issues. You never see a manager doing any clinical care when we are busy. Patients get angry with us and can be abusive. Their visitors and families also tell us off. (B.B., medical staff nurse, 1996)

B.B.'s view of not being able to meet her patient's needs, the complaints by patients, and the lack of concern by management, were echoed by most of the nurses whom I interviewed. Another nurse communicated the following regarding abuse:

> There is abuse from families, verbal mostly. Then they go to the President and he along with the Patient's Rep want to know if we are the guilty party and did we cause this. They want us to put up with anything and treat the patient like a customer. There is no support from managers and we need

to be more assertive. There is far more violence toward nurses in hospitals today. (N.L., orthopaedic unit, 1994)

Most staff nurses lack the time and the energy to deal with abuse and violence that is directed towards them. The staff nurses' dual roles of providing care and also information around care puts them under tremendous pressure. In addition, the nurse has to continue to provide care to individuals who have abused them, or who lodged a complaint against him/her. It has become difficult for the staff nurse to live up to patients' and their families' expectations. There is a pull between quality care versus emergencies that occur on the unit every day, such as a cardiac arrest or a "patient going flat," as well as less staff to do the same, or increased workloads. Added to this are the education sessions that nurses must attend in order to keep themselves current, when policies and procedures are changed. During the time of team conferences and educational sessions, the nurses working on the unit have even less staff to meet patients' needs. Staff nurses have been told by family members that they "would be sued" or that they have "a poor attitude." These threats only add tension to an environment where the nursing care delivery system is strained to its limits.

O.S., a staff nurse, stated: "Usually it is something they want from the hospital or the doctor. We get the family members yelling at us about care, while we are doing our best." Nurses have indicated that they have been physically pulled, called names, and at times hit. The violent behaviour of patents against nurses in the workplace is more common than supposed (*Registered Nurse*, February 1990). Nurses reported that there is a tendency to blame the victim for having caused the violence. Of reported assaults against nurses, 5% cent of the victims were rendered unconscious, 10% had fractures, 21% had life-threatening injuries, 26% had lacerations, and 36% had bruises (1990, 42). Nurses have reported to me that they have been slapped by patients, had urine thrown on them from a urinal, been stabbed, or hit by a walking cane:

> I was hit in the eye by a patient. We had to call security. He was also attacked. He came at me from behind for no reason. We are getting violent patients and even though we get together and write to administration and to the doctors, we still get these patients. I had to be off work for over two weeks. I could be blind... lucky. (V.A., staff nurse)

I had my hair pulled.... I wanted to charge the patient with assault but could not get administration to help me. We have had ten work-related incidents relating to patients and physical abuse and no one will go to bat for us. (P.R., staff nurse, medical unit, 1994)

A patient slapped me in my face, another elbowed me in my ribs. I have been called a nigger, stupid, told to go back to where I come from. One patient told me that he would like to kiss my black lips and even a physician had his hand on my breast. (C.G., medical unit, 1994)

These accounts are not dissimilar to my observation of what can occur on a unit. C.G. informed that she had not reported any of the incidents that happened to her, and that she tried to use humour to defuse some of the situations. V.A., on the other hand, did write to the administration but ultimately "nothing was done." V.A. told me that she felt that "when a problem is about a patient's behaviour no one wants to look at it" and "they turn their eyes." She expressed anger but needed "the job." These illustrations about the abuse that nurses have experienced are similar to the cases analysed by the RNAO (1990).

Abuse between nurses can be traced to the grumbling atmosphere (Mackay 1989, 98) among nurses as early as the 1650s (Bingham 1979). Nurses on night duty have complained to me in interviews, just as is reported by Mackay (1989) and much earlier by Ross (1961), that work left undone by the nurses on days caused friction with night-duty nurses. Indeed, work left undone by any nurse is a source of complaint and anger. This anger, when combined with the level of stress on the unit, leads to name-calling or, as Nurse S.T. told me, "talks so rude" and "is so abusive" (1995 notes). Nurses often look at sick leave as "faking injury." Blame threatens the security of a person's job (Ross 1961). This anxiety provokes some nurses to react with hostile words, calling each other names. Nurses have stated to me that they have heard nurses yelling at each other. In one instance, one nurse pulled another's hair (D.N., staff nurse medicine, 1996) and both were dismissed. A blamed person cannot always prove her or his innocence or even know s/he is being reported. A lack of self-esteem, and, by extension, a lack of esteem for colleagues, may exacerbate the atmosphere (Mackay 1989). Ashley (1980) suggests that nurses' hostility to one another is a reflection of misogynistic beliefs about women. Thus, for example, some nurses explain that the "bitchiness" in nursing is the result of women working together, thereby appropriating the attitudes of men who are misogynists (Mackay 1989, 106).

One woman who had spent more than thirty years in nursing stated the following in an interview:

> Merle, why do you think nurses eat their young? I have just hired six new graduate nurses and I will be placing them on the units where there will be complaints that they have "no skills" and that the older nurse are not paid to teach them and will get angry at them. It seems that they like to destroy their confidence. At the end of my career, I can say that nurses eat their young and are not the helping professionals to each other. I feel so sad. The reason I asked this question was that a young nurse came to see me in tears as she had been shouted at in front of a group by a senior nurse because she could not catheterize a patent. The older nurse told her that she was paid as an RN that she should act as one and that she was "not here to baby you." I believe that we nurses eat our young while doctors don't. What is the difference? They welcome the new doctors and treat them as equals. I have heard so many nurses complain about who gets the heavy loads and call other nurses lazy for so many years…We have a week in May that we call Nursing Week to help nursing. We have a tea, promote the profession and what do we do to help come together and be good to each other? (P.M., 1989)

Nurses do discuss "eating their young" and "horizontal" violence, however there is a passive response within the group when it comes to stopping abuse. On the whole, the behaviours described by respondents show that these instances of abuse are verbal, physical, or emotional in nature. Due to issues of abuse, and the many other factors examined in this book, nursing morale in acute care hospitals in Toronto in 1994 was low. The results of the survey show that 43.1% state that morale was low in their hospital; and as shown in the figure below, less than 10% of the staff nurses saw morale as high in their hospitals.

NURSING STAFF MORALE

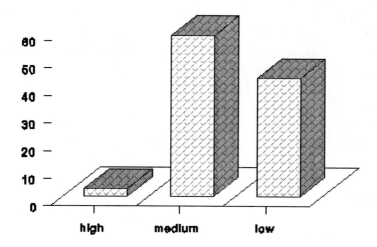

My survey also solicited responses regarding abuse. I found that 87.5% of staff nurses stated that they have been verbally abused by patients, and 62.5% by families. Approximately 52.5% stated that they had been verbally abused by physicians and 34.5% had been verbally abused by other nurses. A total of 47.7% of staff nurses reported that visitors to the hospital had verbally abused them, while 28.1% had been abused by hospital staff. Only 8.6% had been verbally abused by their head nurse/manager. Out of 142 surveys returned, 102 respondents chose to answer the questions on abuse, while between 40 to 62 40 respondents chose not to answer some particular question concerning abuse, depending on the question.

Further, 83.3% of the staff nurses (out of 102 respondents) reported that patients had physically abused them. Only 2.9% had been physically abused by other nurses. Visitors and patients' families were reported by 3.9% of staff nurses as the individuals involved in physically abusing them. Nurses did not report being physically abused by either their managers or physicians. Nurses reported that patients coming out of surgery, or those with brain disorders, would sometimes lash out at them. Many nurses did not define these actions as abuse, but rather saw the incidents as involving patients who were ill, and needed to be restrained, due to the fact that they were not aware of their actions.

On the subject of sexual harassment, only 80 out of the 142 respondents answered the question. In my observation, sexual harassment is not

139

openly discussed by staff nurses. In the survey, 51.3% reported that they had been sexually harassed, while 32.5% of those reported named physicians as having perpetrated the sexual harassment. Another 11.3% reported that a patients' family member had harassed them, while 16.3% reported "other" hospital staff. For 8.8% of the staff nurses, it was their peers who had sexually harassed them.

Only 1.3% of the respondents reported that their manager had sexually harassed them. I am aware that sexual harassment comes in both physical and verbal forms. Sexual jokes at the desk are part of communication that goes on between male doctors and female nurses. Some nurses view this behaviour as sexual harassment, while others view this as "normal hospital" behaviour, and of course for the latter there are limits that are at times crossed.

The male nurses whom I interviewed did not feel that being touched by females on the job amounted to sexual harassment. I have observed male nurses being patted on the behind by their female colleagues and was told by the male nurses: "they meant nothing", and "why get hung up?" So there are varying definitions and comfort levels. As stated earlier, nurses are slow to report abuse, and when it comes to sexual harassment, there appears to be the same or even more reluctance to report these cases.

The culture within the profession is organized in such a bureaucratic manner that it lends itself to rules and outcomes; yet in dealing with abuse hospitals are slow to focus on the abuser when s/he happens to be a physician. Instead, the focus is usually on the victim, who more often than not is a staff nurse. A more appropriate strategy would be to apply policies that are already in place, and lay charges against the abusers. The lack of support by administrators leads the staff nurses to spend energy on getting their complaints heard, usually through their union. Unless reported, the ONA cannot intervene and provide systems that can change this aspect of the culture. The ONA has the ability to censure hospitals that have unsafe working conditions, and hence, nurses need to take an active role in stopping behaviour that is abusive by reporting incidents to their union.

Nurses can report those professionals who are abusive towards them to the respective colleges, as this behaviour is not accepted either by the College of Physicians and Surgeons or the CNO. Within hospitals, there is also the Occupational Health and Safety Committee, which looks at unsafe working conditions. Until nurses report incidents to the appropriate authorities, the abuse that is currently occurring will most likely continue. Racist

140

remarks have been considered in the above section when discussing verbal abuse, and in the next section, the issue of racism in nursing proper is addressed.

Racism in Nursing and the Effects on Nursing Culture

Racist attitudes are manifested within nursing in many different forms. Incidents are perpetrated both by employers, and patients. Minority nurses have described incidents that have been verbal in nature. Personal accounts from nurses whom I interviewed provided insight into feelings of despair, or reactions that attempted to pretend that this behaviour did not amount to "a big deal."

At the unit level, nurses are sometimes labelled by a racial epithet, such as "nigger," by patients. In a committee looking into abuse, a staff nurse stated that:

> A patient called me a nigger and I just smiled at him. I did not report him or respond to him. I don't care what he said because it does not bother me what patients say. I can look after him, and it does not bother me. I just laugh. (M. B., staff nurse, medical floor, 1995)

While this nurse tried to minimize this name-calling, other nurses brought out the point that abuse was not dealt with by those in administration. I found that nurses responded to the verbal racist epithets when they wanted to, if they had the energy to make a complaint, but that most often they avoid the confrontation. Many noted, as well, that a sick person could not be sent home, and that the physician would talk to the patient about the behaviour.

In the area of abuse by patients and visitors, staff nurses felt that most physicians gave them more support than their administrators. Nurses spoke about banning offending visitors, reporting them, or asking someone else to care for the patient when the individual visited. Nurses reported that racist remarks took away from their work, and they had to control their retorts and feelings in order to care for the patient and abide by the standards of the CNO.

As a racialised woman, I have experienced racism. The racism I had believed was occurring for years, but could not account for, became fact when I examined documents received from the hospital and were kept in a

141

secret file. Racism within the nursing profession is identical to that of the larger society, where minorities are asked to wait in line for their turn, or are not given a position because of the colour of their skin. The expansion of equity in society has been slow, and in many circumstances, the law cannot determine the exact nature of the wrong. Social rights are somewhat more difficult to identify. The right to job promotion, the right of racialised leaders to be heard within the profession, the right to share to the fullest extent, and be accorded equal privileges, although all desirable, cannot be guaranteed.

The ONA (in its "Human Rights and Equity: A Guide for ONA Members" document), the RNAO, and the OHA have documented racism that nurses have experienced. The RNAO states:

> Racism is systemic in our society and endemic in our insti-
> tutions. Racism has the effect of excluding groups of people
> (based on their race, colour, nationality, ethnic or ethno-reli-
> gious origin) from decision-making processes and leader-
> ship and economic opportunities. Racism is both an attitude
> as well as the specific actions resulting from that attitude.
> (2002)

Nurses continue to say that racism has a negative impact on the health of individuals (Hagey et al. 2001) and the nursing profession (Duffin 2002). Nurses encounter racism from multiple sources, including clients and their families, colleagues (nursing and others), and the very systems and struc-tures within the workplace (2002, 2). Black nurses in Ontario experience both overt and covert forms of racism (Das Gupta 1996). Although not openly discussed, minority nurses talked about being left out and held back within the profession. They talked about being excessively monitored and marginalized. Minority nurses also described how they are pulled aside and spoken to more often then their white counterparts.

Another aspect that nurses discuss is the "way they speak." Language issues become a part of how they are assessed. Even though they have the educational standards from their own country, the same level as those trained in Ontario universities, this training is viewed as inferior. An example of this occurred when a census was taken at one of the hospitals regarding university degrees. Nurses from Asia with degrees were told that they would not be counted when tabulating the number of professional nurses with degrees in nursing. These nurses spoke about feeling marginalized and contacted the CNO regarding their degrees. Several of these nurses had studied in the United States at the Masters level and knew that their degrees had been accepted in North America. Nursing administration refused to consider their degrees, and it was only by protesting this action, both by calling the CNO, and by being outspoken, that the nursing leadership decided to include the nurses from Asia in the count.

There is silence around racism in nursing. As a minority nurse, I did not hear about racism from other minority nurses until I started this project in 1988. I was told by a Korean staff nurse that one of the reasons I was not at the top of our profession was "because of the colour of my skin." This opened up a discussion in which I learnt that many younger minority nurses saw a barrier that did not allow them to reach their goals. They did not see role models from their own background in nursing, and felt oppressed by management who are mostly white. The 1991 Census indicated that visible minority nurses in Ontario have half the chance of their non-racialised counterparts to move into the managerial level. Although there are minority nurses at the staff level, it is narrow at the top with few visible minority nurses in leadership positions. Racialised staff nurses pointed this out to me over and over again, which led me to label this issue as "the Cappuccino Principle."

To make waves about the issue of racism within nursing is to become labelled as a troublemaker; yet, racism is visible at the hospital level, as well as within the CNO, the RNAO, and the ONA. The patterns are much like those in society, and racialised nurses talk about tokenism, denial of promotion, work allocation, targeting, and excessive monitoring (Das Gupta 1996).

In a case against a hospital in 1998, a nurse was asked by the mediation judge if she would settle the Human Rights action if the hospital would allow her to come in and educate the younger staff nurses around the issues of racism and abuse. Although the nurse agreed to this action, the hospital refused to co-operate. Other hospitals have been asked in the past by the Ontario Human Rights Commission (OHRC) to provide diversity training. As one nurse told me:

I think this issue has been beaten to death. I think that the issue of discrimination is valid in any situation in any job in the world. People still think that nurses are handmaidens and servants in many areas. They will talk behind their back and never resolve the issue at hand. I can't help it if I am white, but I feel that visible minorities are responsible for their actions as I am for mine. (A.K. medical unit, 1995)

The OHA encourages equity and diversity training; however, biases and negative judgements are experienced in the same context of systemic racism that exists in society at large. Immigrant nurses of ethno-racial minority groups have filed grievances about work-place racism. The authors of this report state that:

> Racism as a phenomenon is poorly understood within the profession. Visible minority nurses experience racism in their workplace. With the economic downturns racism will be more rampant (Head) that will bring undue hardship to many visible minority nurses. (Collins et al. 1999)

It is evident that racism is part of nursing, yet nurses themselves are generally silent about this and the hospital environment supports this behaviour. Das Gupta (1996) contextualizes everyday racism in hospitals, and views it in the context of systemic racism in the employment system. Following this work, Hagey et al. (2005) links poor health to racism and points to how nurses are "set-up" due to racist practices. Nurse leaders point to anti-racist policies but do not use the word racism. Another form of racist behaviour practiced by the dominant group within the profession is that the European roots of nursing are celebrated, leaving out the rich history of Black nurses in Canada since 1944. Rather than use the words "race" and "ethnicity," the word that is most often used is "diversity."

Culture competency is also another way to get around dealing with racism within the nursing profession. When we look at nursing in Canada the hierarchical structures are caste-like, reflecting a mirror image of society. White women control nursing and sustain their power through subtle racist behaviours. As observed in a recent study:

> Accreditation in Canadian nursing schools is silent about problems of racism in nursing education, health care and society. Moreover, faculty who break the silence on racism in nursing continue to be marginalized, problematized and contained, i.e., racialised. (Hagey et al. 2005)

Canadian human rights legislation does not stipulate that intent must be proven, allowing that racial discrimination can occur without intent.

The Cultural Value Support and Caring

Another nurse who helped her and wrote to the manager that they wanted a 'code white' for help when they were in danger supported the nurse who discussed the issue of being hit in the eye. Nurses banded together and pushed for the physician to get involved. They gathered money and sent flowers for the nurse while she was on sick leave. Most nurses when talking about "their unit" and the nurses they work with, describe this type of caring and support. I found that I received support from other nurses in the hospital when I was terminated from my position as a nurse manager. I found that minority staff nurses reached out to me, and identified with the issues of unfairness.

Caring and support can be observed in the doing of tasks. Nurse O.N. told me that she liked picking up after her peers in order to help them and would always check their IVs when she was doing hers. She said: "I come in early to get my work in order that I can help some of the other staff" (O.N., interview, 1996). Although staff nurses complain about each other, they help each other when patients are in acute situations, as they do not want errors to occur that would endanger patients. Nurses bond over the issue of good patient care, and for many staff nurses, this is seen as a helping culture at the unit level. As one staff nurse informed me, "we get along better on our unit and help each other" (O.S., interview, 1996). At the unit level nurses take time to help each other with patient care and with problem solving, especially in the absence of management. It is when they feel threatened by new BScN graduates that experienced nurses fall into the pattern of "us" and "them" instead of helping the new staff, as described earlier. This pattern of helping can also be seen in other areas of staff nurse interaction.

When working on projects, staff nurses work well together. Staff nurse V.D. provided the following:

Four staff nurses worked on a medication system plan to help staff cut down on errors. We did not point fingers and did not accuse but looked at why we were making them. We looked at ten errors, discussed the merits of a computer

145

program to help that was patient centred. We wanted a new system.

There are many incidents that staff nurses have reported where they have worked together to plan patient care and to find the right bed for a patient. Transferring a patient from one unit to another requires co-operation among nurses, for example, a co-operative attitude provides for a collaborating culture.

Nurses also state that they have been helped by peers when a physician has shouted at them or when they have been abused verbally. Staff showed support for each other when a physician refused to sign an order and threw a chart across the desk. A letter was written and signed by four staff nurses. They told me that they had concerns about how the physician had "thrown the chart, as he walked out." The lack of respect for their colleague was the greatest factor in their taking up this issue. The nurse said she felt support but was disappointed by administration because they did not respond or make the physician apologize. In their discussions with me several staff nurses informed me that if left alone to work with each other they would have a unit that worked "well, in a team and with respect."

Time off work is another area where staff nurses show how they interact with each other. Nurses have communicated to me that although they have some problems, they share vacation time, trying to make sure that a peer gets some prime vacation time. As E.S. stated, "it is not hogging all the summer weeks." When asked to change shifts, nurses have stated to me that when allowed by the manager, they do find a peer to help them switch their days off. Scheduling time off is difficult for nurses who have a home life and who work full time. Yet, when able to change their shift to help another nurse, my observation has been that staff nurses do help their peers when possible.

When dealing with scheduling problems, E.S., a staff nurse reported that:

> I got a call from a physician demanding to know if the unit had a drug. When told to follow procedure, he called me rude and hung up the phone. The other nurse supported me and we wrote a letter about the physician's behaviour. (E.S., interview, 1991)

146

Staff nurses 'circle their wagons' around a peer when abuse occurs, and when dealing with physicians; there is recognition that it is only when nurses join together that they are able to have a stronger voice. My observation has been that when one nurse goes against a physician, the administration can allow the incident to slide. On the other hand, when a group of nurses take the issue to their manager, and speak out against an issue or incident, some action is usually taken, even if only to acknowledge that an incident has occurred.

Nurse T.L. (1990 notes), in discussing her peers, found that most of them thought her to be a "good nurse." She mentioned that she could rely on them and that she did not have to ask for help. She also explored with me the notion that nurses care for each other, by calling when they are on sick leave, sending flowers, or listening when the other has problems. I know of a nurse who thought all her colleagues on the unit were her friends and had them all to her home for a potluck dinner. Another nurse, O.D., told me that once a month they all go out as a group and have a fun evening. This outside work socialization provides staff nurses with interactions that provide a bond that continues in the workplace. Social activities create an environment in which nurses relax with each other, and get to know each other outside of the hospital environment. When they were able to bring this atmosphere back to the unit, the nurses informed me that they felt much closer, "like a family." As the group interacts during lunch, or outside of working hours, they form a cohesive group.

This same nurse also reported that A.J., another nurse, had to stay late and help the oncoming shift because the Admitting Department had sent the paperwork late. This thoughtful behaviour was noted by E.S. "...as kind and helpful to both staff and patients." Nurses complement each other, and acknowledge when a peer goes out of their way to help. Staff nurses in their discussions reported incidents where nurses have good skills, and helped other nurses. Being supportive and caring are qualities that staff nurses value in the nursing profession.

Both caring qualities and the "bitchiness" are part of the culture in which staff nurses work and socialize. What behaviour occurs in an interaction depends on the relationship of the individuals, the power structure, the hospital culture, and the activity of work at the time the interaction occurs. In emergencies, nurses tend to pull together, and work for the benefit of the patient. I have been informed that those thought to be less competent can be told what to do in emergencies. In non-emergencies, however,

147

those who are considered less competent are gossiped about, and can be treated in a negative manner by a peer.

For many nurses at the staff nurse level, the stress of the job brings out negative reactions towards their peers. A nurse informed me that she felt pulled in all directions, and when someone left work undone she wanted to scream as it meant that she would have to pick up the work. "It is not that I scream, but I feel so stressed." They are short staffed, and at times snap at each other when a stressful incident occurs. This behaviour gets far more attention than the actions of caring that have been described in this section.

During this research, I became aware that nurses addressed negative experiences when asked a question, but when completing the survey, staff nurses gave positive responses about their peer interactions. The question of caring could have been sidelined when dealing with abuse, bitchiness, and racism. The latter are issues that cause problems for staff nurses, and therefore come to the researcher's attention. Caring does occur, however, and is a positive influence on the environment in which the staff nurses do their work.

What is the Culture of Nursing

Staff nurses view nursing as a caring and supportive environment when it comes to the unit where they work. Most of the time they have good stories to tell of how they were helped. As M.P. stated:

> I've seen nurses work together. There are many times when I have seen staff nurses do things for each other that is beyond what they have to do. It is all the other things, like the hospital cut backs, the management, and the change in patients. No longer can we give to our patients as we used to. Our loads are heavy and we are always on the run. But we do have a closeness with each other, although not like we did, it is so busy. I think when something happens we do see the caring for each other, maybe like any other business. Perhaps we think that as nurses we must do more but we do give to each other. Hey we are female and do talk about our emotions and problems with each other but not all the time. Support is still there. (medical staff nurse, 1996)

148

Staff nurses are very much involved in the culture of nursing by their expectations of what makes a good nurse. Their ideals of support, training, and caring are part of nursing culture within hospitals. There is a culture of support which is high when nurses have problems with physicians and when general problems occur. This supportive value is viewed when illness occurs and when staff nurses are allowed to work on unit issues.

When looking through the lens of caring, the profession of nursing within Toronto does not have this value as the core of the profession in the way that it did in the past. It is the ideal of professionalism that has become the core value of the professional culture as provided through the structure of nursing. The ideal nurse for the staff nurse is one who is a supportive nurse and is a team player, whereas the management class in nursing wants the ideal nurse to include an education in which nursing is research-based. Although caring is part of this ideal nurse, it gets lost in the quest for professionalism. This culture is the product of not only a historically based profession, but also of one controlled by physicians and administrators. Through their power over time they have been allowed to foster a verbally abusive culture. As restructuring has occurred and patient care reduced, nurses have experienced an increase in physical, emotional, and verbal abuse from patients and their visitors. Verbal and emotional abuse has also come from peers, which has thus led nurses to coin the term "horizontal violence." "Eating our young" is another way nurses talk about the abuse that goes on with new graduate nurses who need support and mentorship of senior nurses.

According to research studies (Head 1985; Calliste 1993, 1995, 2000; Das Gupta 1996; Collins et al. 1999; Jacobs 2000; Hagey et al. 2001, 2005), racism is exacerbated in periods of economic downturn and has become more acute due to social dynamics. With the increase of visible minorities in the community and with minority nurses coming out of the Canadian educational system, nursing has not addressed the lack of minorities in senior nursing positions. In the hierarchical scheme of whiteness and otherness there is a continuum, of lesser and lesser privilege and more domination and exclusion from resources and power (Hagey and MacKay 2000). The culture of nursing which produces both conflict and collegiality has within it the value of caring that provides nurses at the bedside the reasons for what they do. Although there are some nurses who believe that patient care can be reduced to a numeric value and an objective standard, the staff nurse still in general views the culture of nursing as one where the

149

core value is caring in spite of the abuse and racism that does exist withi
the profession. This culture promotes diversity yet within the structures c
the profession and work life allows for abuse and racism to exist by no
sanctioning those who are the perpetrators.

The culture of nursing in Toronto is one where staff nurses find th
value of professionalism replacing the value of service and caring. At th
same time nursing has not joined the feminist culture of equality but lean
toward the bureaucratic apparatus where problems of domination are still
focus of tension. Staff nurses within the hospital or through the ONA hav
not focused on this issue, but instead talk about internal struggles betwee
those in power and themselves. Nursing clearly has a bureaucratic cultur
in its method of bringing a certain level of recruitment based on educatio
for important posts. It is also noted that the ideal nurse, who is the profes
sional nurse, depends on both hierarchical authority structures within th
profession and expert knowledge. Organizational control by rules whe
examined unit by unit can be different. Formal rules can be in conflict wit
informal norms of conduct on various units. As a consequence, there ar
many subcultures within the culture of nursing. When constructing
macro-analysis that helps us understand the culture of nursing, the socia
phenomena are built up through a construct where the actor's experience i
part of the overall environment, and not the experiences of the individua
unit.

There are wider social implications when dealing with the issue c
racism within nursing. It is the loss of human and social capital. Attentio
has been paid to the racialisation dimensions of work and their social loca
tions. The challenging process of building a coalition to promote account
ability for anti-racism, anti-discrimination, anti-harassment, employmen
equity, and ethno-racial competencies in nursing needs an ever-widenin;
network of dynamic nurse activists—leaders in their communities and/o
nursing associations—and members of the public. Rather than a hierarcha
model, a consensus-building model when dealing with changes within th
profession should be highly valued by female leaders. Nursing is not
however, an egalitarian profession but rather, is a hierarchical profession
with layers and levels of professional governance.

Chapter Five

Behaviour in Nursing: Collegial and Conflictual

The third conceptualization of collegiality is behaviour by individuals that reflects the essence of complex actions that are shaped by both the structure and culture of the organization. This third element of collegiality not only corresponds to role expectations, but reflects the influence of culture of collegiality and the structure of collegiality. When behaviour is discussed in this chapter, the set of behaviours that Styles (1982) provides to the nursing community are presented as a set of expectations of the profession. My particular interest is in the perception that staff nurses have of each other's behaviour, and their understanding of collegial behaviours in light of restructuring of the work life. Their observations provide for an understanding of collegiality from their awareness.

The relationship between what the staff nurse expects of her or his peers and the actual behaviour can produce, either conflict or collegial behaviour among them. Historical data about a peer is also apart of the expectation that affects behaviour and perception. For example, if I ask a peer to help me turn a patient and get refused repeatedly, not only by the first individual but also by other nurses, I will deduce in my mind that nurses do not help their peers. When a peer helps me, however, I will have a different attitude about the behaviour of helping. Historical experiential data provides the individual with information that allows them to prejudge situations and act and react within this complex environment. Gossip also adds to historical data.

Staff nurses usually need help with turning or lifting a patient. This would be a task. They usually turn to a peer to help them with heavy assignments otherwise know as a "heavy" patient. Process activities are usually coming together to put together a care plan for a patient. This is a written plan and at times left undone. What I am stating here is that there is a ranking of needs, and the "doing for" patients is seen as more important than the process orientated activities. It has been my observation that behaviour such as helping is based on task activities rather than process activities. Another part that helps shape an understanding of nursing behaviour is the analysis on the structure of nursing that indicates hierarchical relationships that have changed over time in how it is expressed. The nature of bureaucratic hier-

archy in nursing although appearing flat hospital organizational designs ha
all the characteristics of hierarchy in how decisions are made. Hospitals i
the past had many layers of management within nursing as compared to th
organizational charts of today that can appear flat but still have far mor
division of nursing tasks. Even within the staff nurse's group, there ar
different levels of status that provide for hierarchical relationships withi
the unit. One example of this is the Charge Nurse of a Unit, or the Tear
Leader of a team. There are mentors, preceptors, and clinical experts. Ther
are other individuals such as Personal Assistants Workers (PSWs) wh
provide nursing care on these units and report to the staff nurse thereb
promoting hierarchical relationships at this level as well. Working within
female-dominated work environment has not changed this hierarchica
bureaucratic behaviour that nurses point to as existing between them an
the primarily male administrators.

Set in this environment, behaviour can produce impersonal relation
ships. Yet, the nature of the work and the history of the profession lends o
women's work should lend itself to more caring and supportive relation
ships. Women's relationships with women can be more emotional tha
men's relationships with men, and therefore can be extremely personal an
caring. Then again, nurses are told by other nurses that when a job is to b
done, personal feelings and emotions should not be part of that job, and tha
objectiveness is an important value. Professionalism, which defines colle
giality, does not define conflict. I find both elements of collegiality an
conflict as behaviours within nursing.

Having identified thirteen behaviours that Styles considered to b
collegial, the preceding discussions on culture have revealed the influence
that effect nursing interactions. The working environments and the experi
ences described in interviews will be examined through the lens of the dat
provided in the thirteen items. Although I dwell on the experiences o
nurses and my observations, in this chapter the experiences will b
discussed in conjunction with the questions put to the 142 survey respon
dents. The thirteen questions can be seen as supportive when carried ou
and non-supportive when dismissed by the staff nurse.

For the most part, nurses communicated to me normative concern
of what counts as "good" nursing practice and of behaviours of which the
disapproved. Items such as respect, help, and exchange will be discusse
one item at a time. These are the positive behaviours. Behaviours such a
reporting and complaining cause a combative environment. Due to th

regulatory nature of the profession, when looking at behaviours it is only the expressed communications (either written or oral) that can be discussed, and not the concealed behaviours that occur. My contention, based on the data, is that staff nurses have more conflictual types of behaviours than collegial types of behaviours.

Another concern is that staff nurses do not communicate with their patients—leaving advocacy to the family—and are now communicating about patients. This changes their role in terms of how they behave around patients, as they are engaging with each other and with other professionals at the nursing station, discussing results and outcomes.

For example: when a patient is admitted to a unit, rather than having the staff nurse co-ordinate the information and care, it is left for the family and patient to find "their nurse", and then to be handed a paper to read, or are told to ask questions of the physician. The PSW complains that the staff nurse "...just likes to sit at the desk, read charts, and look at the computer, leaving the care to us." In view of the last observation, it can be argued that collegial behaviour changes as those who perform care-taking services change. This description, however, incorporates the structures, the history, and culturally specific rules and forms of collegiality.

Do Nurses Treat Each Other with Respect?

Nurses are taught discipline in order to make sure that her or his job performance allows for the enforcement of rules and regulations, so that nursing care can take place in an organized and efficient manner. Respect for physicians, superiors, patients, and peers from the time of Nightingale was part of that training. When students fail to meet the standards of decorum as prescribed by the CNO, the training school, and the hospitals, the student nurse could be terminated from the programme. A code of nursing ethics is part of the educational consciousness nurses obtain from texts and lectures at their training institutions, which reinforces the value of respect. Respect is not only taught but there are sanctions attached to disrespectful behaviour. Rudeness is a complaint made when others think that a nurse has been disrespectful. My observation on rudeness is that it is one of subjective judgment, which has often led to a disagreement where one party states that the other was rude while they were states that she or he was "just making a point," or "being firm."

The characteristics of respect are both verbal and nonverbal. Speaking in a loud voice, being angry, not showing others "courtesy" when answering, hanging up the phone on someone who is still talking would be seen as not respectful or rude by those staff nurses who provided me with data. I have observed nurses complaining about a nurse from another unit who was "rude" on the phone, while they were "trying to make a point" and "she would not listen." In my Collegiality Survey, 6.9% answered that nurses always treat each other with respect, 51.1% of respondents stated that nurses often treat each other with respect. When discussing the issue of abuse, however, 34.4% of these same respondents stated that other nurses have verbally abused them. What do these two answers tell us? Perhaps the nature of respect is more complex and different responses vary depending on the nature of the question. To broaden the understanding on the issue of respect, I reviewed the question in the survey where nurses could write down how they thought staff nurses treated them. Although not all respondents answered this question, when describing in her/his own words as to how staff nurses treat each other during working hours, they used "respect/respectful" in many of their statements. Respondent #106 and #120 stated:

> Most nurses treat each other with respect. Cooperation with physical and problems solving is used on an ongoing basis. Support is given in tough days or situation. (#106)

> I feel we treat each other as equals and with respect. (#120)

Even though I did not use the word "respect" when formulating this question, Nurse #65 used the words "respect" and "help" when responding to this question in spite of the fact that s/he thought that some nurses are "quite unethical maybe due to religion" and did not expand what she means by "religion." "Respect for peers" and "courteous" were the positive attributes regarding peer interaction during working hours. As Nurse #140 stated:

> There is a clearly demonstrated respect for each other as nursing professionals. As individuals and also as members of the health care team. Any problem solving situations that may arise are dealt with by nurses in a very objective and constructively communicative mode.

154

Most of the respondents were talking about their unit and the staff that worked within the unit. But when discussing the "visiting" nurse, respondent Nurse #93 stated that there is a difference with regular staff being treated friendly, while the other nurse is not always warmly received. In my observations, this was an issue constantly discussed in unit meetings, namely, how could make those nurses who came in from the Registry or from another unit feel accepted and as part of the team and not a nuisance. With nurses working full time in a hospital and moonlighting as casuals from a Registry there is less negative behaviour towards the outsider in today's work environment. They are still not, however, part of the unit, and the usual social activities. We must bear in mind that this behaviour is occurring when there is a shortage of nurses, and staff nurses view second jobs as an effective way for an individual to accumulate wealth in a constantly changing system over which they have little input in the changes that come about.

Staff nurses when discussing their peers in focus groups, usually spoke about the non-supportive experiences and "how rude" or "disrespectful," the other nurse has been towards them. When they are not treated with respect, respondents think that "they are treated as rivals, seeking the most coveted position," "complaining about the person who is causing the problem," "cruel," and treat each other "rudely including putdowns." Instances given by staff nurses about incidents show nurses snapping at each other, and being angry on a day-to-day basis. Minority nurses do not think they are treated with "real" respect, as they are over monitored and as previously stated reported on by their white counterparts. Consider the comments mentioned previously when nurses use the word "bitchy" (MacKay 1989), which denoted a mean-spirited negative interaction. Although this word is viewed as a negative epithet by feminists, nurses used this word in focus groups to describe "someone I cannot stand." Prejudice and discrimination maintains a social distance between some white nurses and members of the racialised groups and must be addressed by the OHA, ONA, RNAO, and the CNO in a meaningful way.

Nurses know that normative expectation of their role includes respect. Therefore, the patterns of behaviour in public are formal and respectful among the participants. Perhaps when writing in the survey about a normative behaviour nurses focus on positive incidents but when describing everyday life, they tend to dwell on the problems and the behaviours that they find unacceptable. Most of the gossip that I heard from hospital nurse had less to do with respect, and more to do with aggressive manners and in-group versus out-group behaviour. Those nurses viewed as not being part of the clique could be the target of gossip or other negative behaviours such as targeting. Nursing culture depends on communication both at the patient level and at the professional level. Perhaps the first step is to be prepared to acknowledge the existence of informal relationships affecting the work environment. Next, that cohesion and collegiality are built on the shared sense of purpose and that exclusion and aggression towards a peer has social impacts. Lastly, nurses who are taught advocacy for their patients need to speak out to those in authority instead of mistreating each other. This should not be occasional but continuous helping develop self-respect and social justice.

The Exchange of Clinical Ideas

Collegial behaviour (Styles 1982) includes "the exchange of clinical ideas with each other freely." When asked a question about this, 16.9% responded that this behaviour always occurred. When reviewing the exchange of clinical ideas, nurses overwhelmingly participate in this positive behaviour. Staff nurses state that clinical ideas are the knowledge that they get from journals, lectures, textbooks, and conferences. For them it is important to discuss articles that they read with others to find out new ideas.

When helping each other in patient care issues, nurses do share clinical ideas. This behaviour in not limited to one's own unit, for example when a patient in psychiatry is having chest pains, the staff nurse can call on a peer in cardiology to come and help her or him assess the patient. The reverse is also known to happen. I have observed nurses discussing clinical issues, sharing journal articles, and helping each other in arriving at an understanding of the symptoms of ill patients. Nurses ask those with more experience to come and help them in clinical issues, when they are confused about the symptoms that patients are experiencing. There are occasions when a senior nurse will freely provide information to a junior nurse with a critical patient. Nurses view each other as being "bitchy" when staff nurses in positions of team leader or charge nurse fall back on the authority of their positions to get the work done. In short, staff nurses want autonomy and view "being told what to do" as their place in the nursing hierarchy—at the bottom of professional ladder.

Another area of behaviour is when the talkative types "who cannot control their tongues" and "butt into other people's business" and when told to stay out "complain" about not being treated with respect. Nurses complain about the talkative nurse as not sharing clinical information but gossip. Staff nurses make a distinction between what they view as gossip and when they share clinical information. There are no standards for this judgment but rather a subjective analysis of a peer. The meaning of who gossips and who shares information can be the social relations between peers. The labelling as deviant behaviour has largely to do with the intersections of peer relationships, control and privilege within the group.

Learning to share clinical ideas is part of the students' formal training. Students' discuss case studies in a group when on clinical rotations. They see this interaction as part of being a nurse and the necessity for this behaviour to give "good" and "correct" care to their patients. This provides a collegial relationship when the participants in the sharing experience exchange ideas and data. From the information staff nurses provided during focus groups, they view the exchange of clinical ideas to be a "natural" outcome of nursing care. I have heard negative comments when Clinical nurse experts (CNS) "come on the unit" and "don't know what they are doing." Yet, staff nurses are aware that this nurse (CNS) is there to help them with new procedures and promote excellent patient care. Many staff nurses feel "put down" by these experts, who they complain "do not respect our knowledge." They do not view this nurse as a colleague but as part of the hierarchy.

This discussion does not coincide with the view held by Styles who suggests that "...de-emphasized status differences in responsibility and authority; the task organizes the work; leadership and fellowship fluctuate." Staff nurses do not see this fluctuation nor do they have a sense of shared responsibility, and openness. They view the nursing system as one of hierarchies, and resent their diminished role within the health care team; they also see other nurses having authority over them. These perceptions can cause conflictual behaviours rather than collegiality.

Nurses Report Errors Made by Peers to Management

Reporting on peers was seen as negative behaviour. Some nurses in the study compared themselves with physicians who rarely reported on each other, and questioned the difference in reporting behaviour. Both physicians and nurses have a reporting mechanism from their colleges to report errors, and hospitals also have the same reporting system for both professions. It is the nurse who is most often the reporter, however, and it is the nurse who most often gets reported.

From my observations, there are several explanations for the difference in reporting behaviour. A physician provided the first reason when he informed me that physicians were self-employed, and had to look after themselves. If they started to report on someone then they could in turn be reported on, making it difficult for them to earn a living. Therefore, it was important for physicians to support each other, as what happens to one could turn around and happen to another in their group. Self-interest and survival were factors that kept physicians from reporting each other. On the other hand, nurses are employees of the hospital, and are responsible to the institution for their survival.

Status and power provide a second reason that can account for the different response to errors. Physicians have power and recognition, while nurses are still struggling to be recognized as a profession. In my observations, physicians were looked up to as gods, and still get annoyed when their "orders" are questioned. As described in chapter three, the role of the nurse is one where her or his patient is their reason for employment, they take orders from physicians, and errors affect patient care. Given this role, and the work overload due to cutbacks, the majority of patient care errors are nursing errors. When an error is found in a physician's order, usually it is "caught" by a nurse, and the error does not occur—the physician can change the order to the correct one, making it a "potential error". Reporting of errors usually falls onto the nurse who finds the mistake. This behaviour brings out resentment in staff nurses when "a finger is pointed at them." As staff nurse D.C. (1996) told me that she is always checking up and trying to point out errors:

> Some are just signing off orders that we forget. She can call you but likes to report you to the manager. When she makes a mistake, she does not like you to even ask her. Miss Perfect. I got her but good with one of her errors and reported her to the manager. I really can't stand her.

D.C. is not unique in her response, as when discussing reporting behaviour several nurses have described peers in a negative tone and expressed wanting to "get back" at the reporter. This behaviour of reporting is about public safety in hospitals, yet provides for a culture of conflict within the staff nurse group. Nurses discussed "reporting" as communication about performance that goes on initially without their knowledge, with the manager being informed, or an 'incident form' made up about the incident; lastly, the staff that made the error is informed as to what occurred. Reporting errors is different from discovering an error and helping a peer with the error. Most nurses like to report their own errors to their charge nurse/manager or the physician in order to correct the error, and provide good nursing care.

Measuring performance is important, however, it is the sanctions that are questionable. Consequences for errors differ from hospital to hospital. In one hospital, the Director of Nursing Practice came up with a policy "that after four errors the nurse would lose her job." This individual wanted to exercise her power and authority using patient safety as an excuse. Such nurse leaders enforce oppressive practices upon other women with less power. They use standards evoking concern for "best practice" while in reality they are constructing an oppressive culture which allows them power and role importance. Imagine having the power to prevent another woman from working and providing for herself. Rather than re-education and up-skilling, this director wanted to use a recourse that focused on failure rather than access to education. Unfortunately, this director is connected to the elite nurses and such conflictual behaviour is not viewed as problematic. I state this as some errors were as trivial as not completing the Narcotic Form by leaving out the physician's name. The punitive attitude has been an attitude that points to an abuse of power. There are some in management that view errors as a learning experience and treat errors as an organizational problem rather than just an individual's fault. In this way, results can involve changes in policy with educating the individual in how best to carry out patient care.

The reporters of nursing errors, for their part, maintain that they are protecting patient care, as declared by the CNO in their standards of practice. Most nurses with whom I have spoken consider catching errors that affect patient care as a positive action. They do voice resentment around reporting of paper work, minor errors, and writing them up because they missed "signing off" on physicians' orders without first talking to the nurse involved. "Signing off" refers to a nurse checking to indicate that a physician's order was done.

Many nurses complain that rather than calling them to find out if the order was done, there are staff nurses "who like to make trouble for others." In the Collegiality Survey, 50% of the nurses in the survey thought nurses reported errors made by peers. Racialised nurses report that they are targeted for minor errors, while white nurses get away with the same mistakes. They view this as racism within nursing. In the matter of terminating nurses after "four errors," racialised nurses described the director who wanted this policy as a racist who was also an abusive individual. They reported her as shouting at them, and *infantilizing* them for minor issues. Although she had no credibility with them, there was a dilemma concerning what action could be taken regarding her abusive behaviour. Nurses informed me that they celebrated when she left the hospital to take a position at a university. This example shows a lack of accountability of nurse leaders, as well as powerlessness within the staff nurse group.

Hospitals have manual directives in their policy regarding the reporting of incidents that occur on the unit, and the forms contain an area for reporting errors, or potential errors. It is the reporting of potential errors that provide for the major concern among staff nurses. In discussions with me, the majority of nurses felt they were open to comments, and constructive criticism. They want any errors they make to be handled professionally and for interventions to occur between the individuals.

Many staff nurses think that adverse situations are remembered by the individual, because it is traumatic when you first know that an error has occurred and has been reported, is when you are called in by a manager. They report feeling guilty, or upset that an error was made that could cost good patient care. The threat of being reported to the CNO is also a stressor that many discussed during interviews. There are managers who rely on "sneaks" to report on their peers, thus contributing to an environment that feeds conflict. The fear held by some nurses is that some of their peers could try to shift responsibility to another nurse to avoid difficulties themselves. One nurse describes the situation as "a feeling that you are on your own". While knowing one's mistakes helps improve work performance, in some cases it seems to be motivated by punitive goals.

Many nurses in this research agree with the following feelings as stated by Nurse #69, who also wrote in the survey that the morale in nursing is "rock bottom." The nurse stated: "It depends on the type of nurses you work with. If they are helpful and work like a team with everyone else then it is great, otherwise you're on your own."

Sometimes friendship intervenes between making a report and not making one, as Nurse # 129 stated: "Some of the staff nurses treat each other like friends. Some of them treat each other like enemies." Apart from the issue of friendship, race has played an issue in who gets reported. When dealing with the culture of reporting, I was told by a minority nurse that white nurses reported more on black nurses and this nurse felt that race played a role. Along with the race comments comes the issue of friendship and "who is a friend of whom" and "how the team works."

Staff nurses want to feel safe with their peers, and want to know if they can trust them. Such comfort would allow for staff nurses to treat each other in an approachable manner. Error reporting is a common behaviour in hospitals, and for minority staff, it is even more problematic. Those who are not part of the 'in group' on the unit get reported more often, while those who are friends cover for each other. A total of 16% of nurses in the survey thought nurses had rarely been reported by their peers. Perhaps this data highlights "friendship" behaviour. All nurses in the survey said that nurses had been reported by their peers to management at one point—there was 0% in the "never" column—and so there is not one nurse who believes that "nurses never report errors made by peers to management." Nurse #51 stated that she found nurses to be "quick to criticize any errors or short comings, and are more easily in Labour and Delivery than in Psychiatry. As stress and overwork increase, so does conflict between nurses."

Reduced staff levels, the type of unit culture, stress, and overwork were reasons provided by staff nurses as to why their peers were quick to criticize. When management approved of the reporting of non-threatening errors, this culture empowered those individuals in nursing who were "quick to criticize any errors or short comings", rather than contributing toward a learning environment. When discussing the reporting errors between nurses, there is a structural base that requires this behaviour, due to public safety accountability through the CNO. The management of errors is different from reporting errors. How an error is managed will either provide for a learning environment, or a punitive environment. The type of culture relating to errors is far more unit and hospital based. A culture that encourages reporting on peers also provides fertile ground for complaining behaviour, as we will now go on to discuss.

Nurses Complain to Peers when Talking About Work Habits

In Style's view, "remediation, rather than blame setting or blame avoid ance," is collegial. In the Collegiality Survey, I looked at the act o complaining, which is indirect and blame setting, in order to examine behaviour that compromises and negotiates in such a way that it can b viewed as blame avoidance. Complaining behaviour, like reporting behav iour, increases conflict among nurses. The ramification of this behaviour i a breakdown in collegiality. Complaints from one nurse about another car range from "not helping a patient look for hearing aid batteries" or "did no get an interpreter for a patient" to more patient-care issues such as "unpro fessional, she leaves the patients with their meals unfinished." When asked if the individual had voiced her complaints to the nurse she wa: complaining about, she informed me that she had spoken with other staf and that they all felt the same way about the issues. She called it "sharing" and "finding out" what other's thought about the problem.

When discussing this issue with staff nurses, I found that staf nurses either did not like to confront each other or be direct. Nurse D.C (1997) stated that she found that "nurses gang up on one individual" anc "rat on her to the manager, you would think that they would have cama raderie." When talking with groups of staff nurses, they would lead the discussion to complaining about the nurses' patient care decisions that occur under the guise of improving patient care. Competence is the main subject area that nurses like to complain about when talking about othe staff nurses and the way they behave. They weigh clinical experience, judg ments, and the proper level of accountability in the discussion of work habits. Due to the fact that the staff nurses' physical environment is oper for all to observe, conduct is judged and discussed. Complaining to each other and gossiping about errors were similar behaviours for some nurses in this research.

The above three behaviours—complaints, blame, and gossip—are most often viewed as negative by staff nurses. This does not mean that the three behaviours are identical but that they support the idea that respon dents have reported that staff nurses treat each other "badly," "mean-spirited," or "bitchy."

Nurses complain about the government, the hospital, the profession and other health care providers as well as their peers. When a fifth of the respondents stated that staff nurses always complain, it raises questions

162

about a work environment that allows for this behaviour. Perhaps errors and problems are introduced as specific reasons for these behaviours; staff nurses think that they do not always get blamed or gossip when they make errors. S.N. (1997, medical unit,) when discussing the three behaviours listed above, described complaining as nurses talking to each other, while blaming was pointing a finger. Gossip was close to complaining but had a more negative connotation.

Reviewing my three survey columns (always, often, sometimes), I found that 92.3% of the respondents saw other nurses complaining, 86.2% found them gossiping, and 76.9% thought blaming occurred. Blaming behaviour is the least liked of the three behaviours and appears to be seen the least by the respondents. In the survey, more than 20% think blaming behaviour rarely occurs. Some nurses have learned to account for blaming behaviour when problems arise, as well as the checking up on peers and the reporting that occur among some nurses. In interviews and group discussion, staff nurses resent being blamed for errors. In my survey, 76.9% of the 142 respondents have seen blaming occur at least some of the time.

Gossip is another behaviour that has been reported as negative. Several staff nurses have communicated to me that they did not want to "get involved," "socialize," or "become friends with" nurse X because she or he gossiped. "Complainers" as some nurses are called by their peers can be informed that they are complainers and "to stop as no one wants to listen" to them (V.D. 1996). In my observation, complaining is more accepted than gossiping or blaming behaviours. Although several nurses have told me that they would like group solidarity, they have also stated that the three behaviours discussed in this section do not allow for group solidarity to take place on an ongoing basis. Informal groups arise spontaneously when crises occur which are supportive, and when there are groups of nurses on each unit that are supportive of each other. I add here that staff nurses do negotiate with each other, and also provide feedback to each other. These behaviours come from assertive nurses who feel empowered by their knowledge and skills.

Nurses Encourage Peers in Risk-Taking Behaviour

Risk-taking is a positive behaviour that Styles (1982) saw as collegial; that is, in creative problem solving, challenging oneself, or thinking beyond the limits of one's role. In hospitals, the risk management programmes are in place to help minimize the risk of liability. The nurse is exposed to risks that occur by virtue of the nature of service they provide. In order to take risks, staff nurses would have to have a safe environment where they would know that they would not be constantly liable, complained about, or gossiped about. Many nurses have voiced concern over the potential conflict surrounding risk-taking behaviours as it relates to change. Unfortunately, tensions from restructuring and downsizing exacerbate perceptions that there can be consequences for risk-taking behaviour. Therefore, the results in the last section (complaining, blame, and gossip) provide another perspective into understanding that collegiality among nurses be limited because the culture does not permit for this to occur.

Recognizing that racism is part of nursing culture, the ONA provided workshops for staff nurses (*ONA News*, October 1994) on dealing with racism, discrimination, and employment equity. Staff nurses do not grieve or use the Human Rights process because they do not want to "rock the boat." However, black staff nurses have told their stories of how white peers within the ONA have pushed them out of office or not involved them in meetings. Minority nurses were over-monitored and targeted. Risk-taking behaviour becomes a stressful event. No matter what the outcome was, comments from white nurse managers of how it "should have been done" were common when it came to racialised nurses.

Several ethnic minority nurses also described how they were targeted, and this knowledge made them concerned about their job. Describing their experiences and frustrations even though represented by a union, nurses felt that systemic racism and discrimination was impossible to prove. Additionally, they commented on the fear that when there is a shortage of jobs they would be the first to be unemployed or underemployed. This fear would make them double-check their work and not take risks. Therefore, racism and abusive behaviours provide a culture that does not support risk-taking behaviours for many minority nurses, and encourages staff nurses to be followers rather than risk-takers. White nurse managers speak about social justice, accountability, and advocacy yet do not put into practice what they espouse. Perhaps, they see these areas of change for themselves and do not take into account that in leadership roles it is their duty to self examine attitudes, look at behaviours, and suggest steps that transform the system to one of openness and the rejection of racist behaviours. Research (e.g., Hagey et al. 2005) points to racism in nursing and how it should be corrected. Nurse leaders have not taken steps to involve themselves with these changes.

My analysis is that nurses who are complained and gossiped about would be less likely to take risks as they are afraid of the recourse that could occur. The data from the survey shows that 67.5% of nurses think that nurses rarely and never encourage peers in risk-taking behaviour. When discussing this with a group of nurses (focus group, December 1997) they informed me risk-taking has to do with trust. They stated that they had to "watch their backs," that they "could not trust," that "risk taking behaviour was not approved," and that "managers want you to follow the policy." Staff nurses saw risk-taking behaviours as "standing up to unreasonable changes in unit systems." For example, this would be whenever a new director or manager was hired and in order to prove themselves would bring in new systems that did not add value to patient care. This new manager wanted followers, not risk takers. Followers would provide power to the new manager even if it meant more work for them. Another area would be assertiveness with physicians, managers, and visitors who had demands that removed the nurse from the patient's side. They also stated, however, that they did not have the energy to fight the system or make waves, and that they were tired and did not want too many risk taking behaviours.

The following of rules have historical roots in the structure of nursing from the days of Nightingale. Rule following and risk-taking behaviour are not compatible. In my experience and observations, nurses who are strict followers of rules rarely take risk. To improve the care of their patients is a safer arena for staff nurses to take risk. Activities to improve patient care are implemented in committees in most hospitals. I have observed staff nurses participating in committees and providing input. When nurses look at risk-taking behaviours, it is usually challenging in areas that do not affect the well being of patients. This phenomenon has been acknowledged by most of the nurses that I have discussed risk taking with and observed over the years.

Nurses Help Each Other When Problems Occur

In the view of the nurses interviewed, helping behaviour—both in patient care and when problems arise—is seen as an important role expectation. Data from the survey shows 20% of the respondents thought that nurses *always* helped each other when problems arose. Nurses are taught through nursing education (Baumgart and Larsen 1988) that the caregiver role is the most visible aspect of nursing practice. The role lends itself to caring for

165

others and extends itself to helping each other when problems occur. The complex influences of complaining and gossip compete with helping a peer. Clearly the relationships can be considered characteristics of collegial relations when nurses, 70.5%—a majority—think that they are either always or often helped when problems occur.

Nurses have expressed to me that they were helped by another nurse when a cardiac codes is called or when a patient "turned sour" (becomes seriously ill or near death). They also informed me that they could discuss some of their family problems with peers who helped them. The changing of days off was another area that nurses felt that peers helped them with especially when they had problems. On the other hand they also stated that they could not trust all nurses. The helping behaviour tended to be around patient care and shift issues. Nurses informed me when it came to staff meetings, they did not find staff nurses supporting each other on issues against management. For example, on one unit, a staff nurse had discussed "self scheduling" with her peers prior to a staff meeting, yet, when she brought up the issue during the meeting, her peers remained silent. The manager left the meeting thinking that she was the only one who wanted this change. Some nurses commented: "They don't help in the meeting" and "you feel alone".

It appears then that nurses are generally less helpful with each other when it comes to errors, risk-taking behaviour, and complaints. When problems occur on the unit, however, nurses feel that help is available from peers.

Nurses Accept Your Opinion When They Make a Mistake

Data from the survey also provides an understanding as to why nurses report each other and complain about other nurses' work habits. Styles expectation is that "nurses take seriously the opinions of others; hear dissent objectively." The survey data shows over 50% think that they will "sometimes be listened to," and so the behaviours that Styles describes do not always occur among staff nurses. When nurses think that their peers will sometimes listen to them, the question becomes, what should a staff nurse do about concerns? A staff nurse informed me in an interview that she had smelled alcohol on another nurse's breath. This happened over and over again, and she complained to other staff, because she did not know if she could talk to the nurse who was abusing alcohol on duty. In the end, a senior staff nurse informed the manager, and the individual involved was terminated.

Policies and procedures of the institution had mandated that a nurse report suspicions to a supervisor. In the case of a one-time incident, a nurse who accepts another nurse's input can help to learn from the mistake, which can then be corrected. In cases of repeat behaviour, however, many nurses have informed me that they have been accused by the perpetrator of being "a spy" or "the manager's pet" or similarly demeaning slurs. Only 3.9% of nurses think that other nurses accept their opinion "always." Perhaps one of the reasons that nurses gossip, complain, and report on each other is that they are reluctant to voice their opinion to each other as they are not sure of the response they will receive.

The responses to the survey reveals that nurses focus on the negative behaviour of their peers, prompted another area of discussion: why do staff nurses discount the opinion of their peers when they make mistakes? In the discussion of the structure and the culture of nursing, I noted that nursing culture has its roots in the structure of nursing, which then directs nursing behaviours. Nurses have been taught to focus on what they miss, the errors they make, and to catch the mistakes of others, in order to provide a safe environment for their patients. I have noticed in my own training, and also as a graduate nurse that when new student nurses came on the unit, their work was checked for errors by senior nurses. At times praise was also given when nurses provided "good" care for their patients, however, the negative comments outweighed the positive ones.

In a culture where following rules is important, there is an expectation that nurses are there to do a job. Caring for others is also taken for granted, and like mothers in homes, there is an absence of praise and approval given to the caregiver. Therefore, in the absence of praise and approval, it is not unusual for a staff nurse, when asked about negative behaviours, to respond as they did in this survey. In the survey, approximately 15.3% thought that a focus on negative behaviour occurs rarely, and a majority 73.6% responded that they often, or sometimes, thought that nurses focused on negative behaviour. When on breaks and during "chat" sessions, the comments pointed to negative stories, and omissions by a peer.

The focus on negative behaviour, and on not accepting a peer's opinion are behaviours that feed off of each other. It appears that one circumstance gives rise to the next, and is clearly an area where more research is needed. My research and experiences indicate that if nurses

167

thinks that there is far too much focus on negative behaviour, they discount the comments of peers when they make an error, or if in the eyes of 'the other', they have not acted in the best interest of the patient.

Nurses Compliment Peers for a Job Well Done

Nursing culture, with its blaming, gossip, and complaining about each other does not support compliments from peers; yet it does support nurses receiving complements from physicians and patients. Nurses are used to working in a team, whereby they offer assistance and support to each other. When asked about complimenting each other, I was told that they "did not need it", or that they were "too busy to go around making nice." The data shows that 25.3% of staff nurses think that nurses rarely or never compliment their peers. Only 5.4% of this group thought that nurses always complimented their peers for a job well done. Nurses described themselves as not needing to be patted on the back; and one respondent explained that this is so "because we are professionals and are working for the patient" (RN #130).

Complementing behaviour would likely help nurses to create a collegial culture, and so why do they find it easier to blame, gossip, and complain, rather than build up and support each other? When asked "why can't nurses unite?" a staff nurse stated:

> I know my experience is not universal but I have observed and worked with *a number of nurses who haven't learned to care* for themselves. They take 15-minute lunch breaks, take on extra work, do double shifts, and then complain about how they are abused. *Management perpetuates* this by continually asking [demanding] nurses to extend themselves. When nurses assert themselves and point out the reality of the job, *they are called complainers or trouble-makers*. I think there is *real anger* that is harboured by nurses and goes unexpressed until an easy target comes along. It's much *easier and safer to lash out at our colleagues than to honestly assert our needs to management. I think this keeps us disunited* and will be perpetuated this way until we each individually *assert ourselves* and *support our nurse peers* at the same time. In light of the present *economic situation* it's not any easier for nursing to speak

out considering the real risk of losing their livelihood. But I also think that some of us are *more comfortable* to stay *in this position* than to actually rally for change. *Standing up* for oneself takes guts and *puts yourself at risk*, but I think it's the only way for nursing to give itself the empathy and support that we already give our patients. I must admit it is *very difficult for me to fulfill*. (B.C. October 1995).

The statement deals with the lack of positives within the profession. Over the years that I spent talking and listening to nurses, the issues raised in the above statement were voiced over and over again.

In order to give to others, the individual must know how to take care of her or himself. When nurses do not take breaks or work after-hours to finish their work, they put their patients ahead of their needs. Modern feminism has effectually spread the idea that nursing is not only women's work but the work of exploited women. Perhaps it is the feeling of frustration and powerlessness that contributes to the behaviour. In order for the individual to stand up and take risks, the culture for risk-taking must be in place. Positive behaviours such as compliments when they occur get lost in negative behaviour such as blaming and gossiping. Nurses were able to remember and provide me with negative comments or gossip, and could not do so when it came to recalling compliments from peers. On the other hand, they were able to repeat complaints that they had received from patients and physicians.

Nurses get support from their peers when they have problems with Physicians

Physicians have an active role with nurses in the traditional power relationships within the hospital structure. When conflict occurs between a nurse and a physician, 16% of the nurses have expressed the view that administration always sides with the physician (survey question). Perhaps because of the perceived relationship between the administrators and physicians, when problems arise between a nurse and a physician, the nurse is supported by his or her peers. Staff nurses in their discussions with me have related anger, mistrust, and other negative feelings and comments toward the hospital administration. Therefore, rather than negotiating the conflict, nurses take the side of their peer. At least 77.1% (combining the always and often categories) of the respondents thought nurses supported each othe when problems arose with physicians, while almost the same percentag found that administrators sided often/sometimes with physicians.

It appears from the research that the negative attitudes are trans ferred towards the physician, and nurses take sides. We can also view nurses' support for peers as coping mechanisms in a bureaucratic organize tional culture. It can be suggested that they support each other because the work as colleagues on a daily basis, and thus understand the problems tha occur on the units. There has not been any effort that I have observed tha pulled staff nurses together when one of their peers has been in conflic with the administration.

This is exemplified in an incident that occurred in the late 1990 and was reported on in the local media. What occurred was that a group c nurses complained to the Human Rights Commission about the racisr within their hospital. They found it difficult, and requested help, not from their own nursing union but from the Ontario Federation of Labour (OFL) With the help of June Vicock, this was the first case that was settled. Th OHA responded in 1996 by providing a video to hospitals concernin racism.

Abuse, Harassment, and Racism

Abuse is overt and is discussed by staff nurses over coffee breaks and a lunch; however, harassment and racism are spoken about far less ofter Nurses reveal what others do to them but do not always mention what the do to each other. Several nurses were open in their discussion of this issue Nurse C.M. said that she was told:

> "You are authoritarian and overbearing." I got into an argu-
> ment over how to handle a patient problem. The patient was
> loud and it was past 10 p.m. and other patients were sleep-
> ing. The patient had turned around and hit me and pushed
> me. I asked her to help me settle the patient and she told me
> that it was my fault that I got hurt. (1989)

Faultfinding is a past-time for many nurses. As stated previously, in nursin culture reporting is seen as positive behaviour. The lack of support i evident when racist acts or abuse occur at the hand of a patient or manage

170

ment; and it is different from the support that nurses give each other when the physician is the abuser.

The arguments over working and how nurses should work, provides a fertile ground for conflict, as well as verbal abuse. Nurses have called each other incompetent, lazy, and stupid in my presence. Conflict occurs between those with years of experience and with the "new nurse," and many gossip about what the "new nurse" did not do. I have heard nurses yelling at each other over conflict around "dirty" work.

Many instances were provided to me that demonstrated that nurses felt that they did not act in a professional manner; in most cases, it was the tone of voice or the "telling off" that they labelled as abuse. When mistakes are made and gossiped about on the unit, it comes with condemnation, humiliation, or embarrassment. Some nurses have communicated to me that this behaviour is abusive. They have also pointed out that it fosters a less collective defence among staff nurses than that which exists within the medical staff group.

Another example is that of a Risk Management nurse who reported on a nurse without her knowledge. The complaint was that the nurse should know how to complete the report. She objected to having to go to the unit every time something—such as the record number—was missing from the report. This became an item that was reported to the senior nurse administrator. This culture of reporting on nurses provokes mistrust and anger toward "these paper-pushing nurses." One respondent describes it thus:

> Errors are covered up in the routine of our day when it comes to physicians. But when it comes to us, we have a report to fill in when we find that anything has been missed. I know that some mistakes are more serious, but we have a night nurse and another one on evenings that like to go over all our work and find things out what we have not done. Then she reports it to the manager. I have seen these type of nurses before and they are so evil. Not that they are perfect. I told her off and wrote her a nasty note. All I forgot to do was to sign off an order, which she could do and it was not an urgent order. One time she asked me if I understood English when telling me to do something. (C.C., staff nurse, 1997)

When asked what this behaviour meant to her, she told me that this wa "mean and abusive as well as racist." Three nurses reported on the wa ethnic minorities are treated during orientation: they found that behaviou towards "white" (English/Anglo-Saxon) nurses was friendlier, and tha white nurses were given more time by management and peers to adjust t the unit. The nurses who discussed this were (white) ethnic minority nurse who had observed these behaviours.

Laughter can also be used to belittle a peer. C.M., when discussin; the following incident, found that she felt angry when recalling it. Sh thought the laughter was due to her being black, and that the reaction wa "so rude." It should be noted that "rude behaviour" is how some nurse describe negative behaviour:

> I overheard another staff laughing at me when I stuck my index finger with a needle. They laughed and told me that I did not know how to cap a needle and this is a simple task. (1990 notes)

Needle sticks are a serious concern because of the AIDS virus and othe transmitted diseases, and so this laughter was interpreted as her colleagues lack of concern for her. Clearly, this type of behaviour is characterized a emotional abuse.

Minority staff nurses cope from day-to-day with racist remarks fron visitors and patients who often tell them "to go back where they came from." They find it more difficult, however, to deal with the ones they receive within the profession. A.K., a nurse working on a Medical Unit once came to see me in tears. She told me the following:

> I am accused by another white nurse of not looking after her patients. I feel my manager and a group on the unit do not like me because I am going to university. I think they do not like me because I am black. They go to coffee together and change their coffee breaks to be together and socialize outside. I am not asked to go to lunch with them. They also give me a heavy patient load and the manager gives two nurses in that group extra weekends. (1989)

Staff nurses in other areas also reported what they saw as racist behaviour. The following are two statements around racial tension between whites and non-whites among the staff nurse group:

> There are a lot of problems on my unit. The complaints made are by white nurses against black staff. There is racial tension and I am the team leader. I don't know what to do to help communications. (G.R., operating room, 1990)

> White nurses are not concerned with sickle cell anaemia, and do not encourage physicians to test African and Middle Eastern heritage individuals for this. There are problems between white and ethnic nurses. The white nurses have the ear of the V.P. of Patient Services and the Director of Nursing who both are white. They write their complaints about black nurses in the department. There is one white nurse in this group and she is the one who brings us the news of what the white nurses are saying about us. (H.S., medical unit, 1990)

In my observations, when a minority nurse discusses the issue of racism with her peers, it can be looked at as a non-racist issue but as one of her work life, and nursing life in general. Rarely have encounters between minority nurses helped paint a picture of racism, and of course, added to the picture is the fact that staff nurses believed that their peers targeted them.

As a minority nurse, I found racism to be a subject that was not discussed or dealt with in the open. A black nurse told me the following:

> I overheard some white staff nurses talking about another nurse being transferred to our unit. They were saying that they had far too many of us on their unit, and that they did not want another minority nurse. They were talking about how they needed to talk to the Director and explain that the nurse should not be transferred. I have to tell you that when I first came to this unit they tried to make trouble for me, and I refused to leave. You just have to do your best and then more. They do put minorities in charge at times but look for the most junior in order that they can't be challenged or in order that they can fail. (J.B., staff nurse, 1992)

173

When reviewing the statements, I see the elements of being set-up, being rejected, and having to prove oneself over and over again. Minority nurses find themselves having difficulty when transferred to choice units, such as the Out Patient Departments, or Speciality Units; in addition, they find it difficult to obtain these positions. One nurse commented about this situation:

> I have a lot of experience and courses in this speciality. The first time I did not get a full-time position I was told I did not have qualifications that they needed. This time I did not get the position but found out that a white nurse with no speciality qualifications got the position, and has been working in this area for only two years, while I have been in the area, and in this hospital for over ten years. I am going to Human Rights about this. (L.D., staff nurse, 1997)

Racialised nurses find it difficult to get hired as managers even though they usually have more education when competing for the same position. L.D told me that an 'East Indian' nurse had been hired for a position, along with a white nurse but that the minority nurse had a degree. This discrimination takes place in areas other than hiring. According to my observation, racism also occurs in higher levels of nursing education. Racialised nurses have reported that they find it difficult to attain seats in the MScN program, and also that there was only one non-white student among the twelve students.

I would like to emphasize that not all white women in power are the same, but that there is a group of white women who are dominating the profession of nursing without concern for equity. I was informed that minorities were discouraged, not given the "same breaks" or education dollars within the nursing department at the university. I encountered the "exclusion" behaviour when my nursing peers were given education time to attend university, while this was withheld from me. In fact, I found out that nurses in administration laughed at my achievements, and denigrated my Ph.D.

These nurse leaders have important roles in the nursing profession, yet they do not view their behaviour as dangerous to others, nor do they acknowledge that they create a toxic work environment. Racialised women also told me that nurses studying at university found it difficult to enter the Ph.D. programme. Selection criteria is most often 'who you know', not

174

'what you know'. The slant to give seats to white women, or to give them an advantage, although unsubstantiated, is mentioned by ethnic minority nurses when they discuss graduate studies in nursing.

For example, I was informed that out of three women applying for the graduate programme with the same references, the nurse with an ethnic minority surname did not get a seat. Her two peers, who, on the other hand, had Anglo-Saxon names, were given seats at the Masters level. Prior to applying, the ethnic minority woman pointed out this possible eventuality, and was not surprised when it occurred.

It is difficult to prove when senior nursing managers try to point out that you "lack skill," and twist patient-care issues to show that they have skills while you "lack skills." As a racialised woman, I found myself being called to account for physicians' actions. I also noted that although I was an expert in Mental Health Nursing, the Director of Nursing Practice, with limited skills in this area, constantly questioned my judgment. She did this to empower herself while at the same time controlling and demeaning the other person. This type of set-up, where actions are taken out of context and blame ascribed to the individual, shows how racism can occur under the guise of "quality of patient care". White privilege allows these nurse leaders to hire others like themselves, provide entrance to higher education to those like themselves, and to mentor other white women. These practices continue to diminish opportunities for racialised nurses, and perpetuate racism within the profession.

To try to prove that these behaviours are not only non-supportive but are also racist, and to go against those who discriminate, not only takes time but also tremendous amounts of energy. The nurse has to be prepared to go to court, or to the Human Rights Commission, and to expend both time and money to expose the individuals who have prevented her/ him from achieving her/ his potential. Given their roles, the nurse leaders have hospital lawyers to come to their defence. As mentioned earlier, apart from the legal limits, this type of abuse is similar to domestic violence. As a society we have become more aware of domestic violence, and there is a lack of tolerance for husbands who commit this type of crime. The same intolerance is not present when racist behaviours, bullying, and other forms of abuse occur in nursing.

Analyzing racism 'at the top' is difficult but in speaking to racialised managers and educators like myself, a similar picture emerges. With the distance of time and working in a different profession, I view the behaviours of some administrators, not just as dysfunctional but as racism. As a manager, I found that the Vice-President of Patient Services supported white managers while she targeted me, expecting me to leave and make room for one of her white friends whom she had been trying to hire since her arrival. I was not the first racialised manager that she had targeted. The documents I obtained through my lawyer confirmed to me that she encouraged two members of my staff to report on me. I also found that she encouraged white managers to report to her about their interactions with me; yet she did not ask me for my side of the story.

These kinds of documents help the targeted racialised individual know that they are not paranoid, that they are not dysfunctional, and that they are being systemically disenfranchised. I have been informed by racialised nurse managers that they were terminated by hospitals after being targeted, and that white women where hired in their place (Interviews with BJ, CR, and PM). For example, out of the seven nurse managers at my hospital, the black manager and I were excluded from receiving retention packages that the five white managers received. These funds came out of tax dollars, yet there is a lack of accountability about how these funds are used, as hospitals act like private domains while using public funds. I have been told that this behaviour is not unique to the hospital where I was employed. F.F. and R.M., both nurse managers, told me that as restructuring occurs, the white administration has been able to "push out" minority managers as well as minority nurses. Favouring those who are like you is sometimes conscious, and sometime unconscious. What is assured, is that it threatens the well-being of those who are viewed as "the other", and denies them the same rights and privileges on racial grounds.

Other examples of how racism works include who gets heard, and how complaints are given legitimacy. Staff who complained about what they did not like about my decisions as a manager were given hearings; yet staff complaining about their white managers were silenced and told to speak to their manager and not come to nursing administration. Black and other minority staff nurses reported that they were not heard when reporting a white manager. Racialised nurses point to this kind of racism in nursing that is ignored, or is given lip service treatment by ONA and the RNAO. While Toronto will have more than 50% visible minority citizens by the year 2006, hospital management in Toronto continues to become more white. White nurses hold most of the positions in nursing education, and nursing management in Toronto. To stir this cappuccino needs the help of the OHRC and the government who pays for nursing services and nursing education.

Collegial Behaviour in Nursing

This discussion of nursing behaviour at the unit level refers to that which is observed at the patient level, with peers, and within the hospital team. There is a range of behaviours that occurs and which produces patterns of relationships and interactions among colleagues as they perform their functions. A theme that occurs when observing the behaviour of staff nurses is the significance of nursing culture, in which nurses find themselves. Morale in nursing is not high; only 3.1% of respondents stated that morale in nursing is high, while 43.1% stated that it was low in their organization. Several factors contribute to this low morale; the fact that 61.8% of the nurses responded that they are made to perform non-nursing tasks could be one such factor. Added to this is the increased acuity (sickness) of hospitalized patients, and the changes in communication patterns through changes in technology. The pressures of the current health care environment, and the current changes increases competition among nurses, thereby decreasing collegial behaviour. The set of behaviours that manifest gossip, complaints, reporting, and blaming, provide for a conflictual environment. All of these factors contribute to low morale.

Some staff nurses do interact with each other as colleagues. They view respect and exchanging of clinical ideas as important behaviours; 50% think that these behaviours occur often. Helping is another behaviour that at least 50% of the nurses thought occurred in peer interactions. It is difficult to isolate feelings around gossip and complaining, and how they affect the more positive behaviours of respect, exchanging ideas, and helping each other when problems arise. When working together, nurses express both behaviours at one time or another. The variables of downsizing, restructuring, patient acuity, and job stress influence reactions in any given situation. When discussing the issue of collegiality, staff nurses saw the negative and positive behaviours as associated with women working with each other. Narratives about how "women put other women down" or "women support you emotionally" when statements as to why certain behaviours happen.

What do we understand about collegial nursing behaviour? I see it as a dynamic process and something that is effected by the historical aspects of women's work, the bureaucratic culture of the profession (as discussed earlier), and the health care system. Understanding interaction described by staff nurses helps in the understanding of collegial behaviour which are threatened by the reporting of errors, complaints about other nurses' work habits, the rare encouraging of peers in risk-taking behaviour and gossiping when other nurses have made errors. Perhaps this is due to a attempt to identify with the oppressor and gain management's approval Various minority groups coveted the same praise behaviour, and the compete with each other for status and resources. They align themselve with the organization, and as subordinates, discriminate against each othe in order to gain resources—-these are a few of the ways that the group i power divides and conquers (Neugebauer 1995).

The narratives that have been provided are about a lack of friendli ness due to a lack of positive communication. For these reasons, nurses ar often contentious when communicating with each other, resulting in no supportive behaviours. In some cases, the problem arises strictly out of personality clash. No one is expected to get along with everyone, and thi can be true for the staff nurse as well. What hurts collegial behaviour is pre conceived notions about a peer and consulting with colleagues abou another's behaviour without involving the concerned nurse.

When staff nurses think that there is more negativity within thei peer group, they do not view the group as collegial. When problems occu with physicians, however, nurses find collegial support from their peers The "we" versus "them" behaviour provides for a sense of solidarity amon the group when conflict or problems arise. Understanding relationship between members of a professional group comes through understanding th behaviours as they connect with one another. I can state that the relation ships are wide in range with both obstructions to collegiality on one hand and good communication among staff nurses on the other. Nurses do no appear to be apathetic towards each other. Closeness also arises out o friendships and helping each other with psychological issues such as birth and deaths; however, collegial behaviours doe not necessarily mean friend ship. There is a collaborative relationship around patient care, but a absence of a total collegial relationship as advocated by Styles. While ther is a general perception from staff nurses that there are more negative behav iours when interacting with each other, they are aware that associated witl their interaction is a team approach with respect, support and a perceivec understanding of the other's struggle and accomplishment.

178

Collegial behaviour occurs when staff nurses take the time to listen to concerns and provide helpful information to each other. While the nurse usually takes the brunt of difficult situations she or he does not have to deal with it alone. Drawing on support from each other by sharing clinical ideas, nurses know they "provide good patient care." All nurses interviewed for this project agreed that even the most collegial peer could have "her days." When he or she has one of these days, nurses try their best to explain it away. In conversation after conversation with staff nurses working in Toronto, it became obvious that the issue of clinical practice was an important issue in the face of health care restructuring. Fear of job loss and underemployment as well as having to do more with less was more stress than they could handle. Behaviour also depends on attitudes, and one respondent's questions can be seen as such an indicator. The following questions were asked by D.R. (October 1995) when discussing the profession:

> Why are nurses weak?
> Why do doctors have all the control?
> Why can't nurse unite?
> Is solidarity a term to be reserved for unions only?
> Why do we eat our young?
> How do we change all of this?
> Why are we being replaced?

All of these questions look at the negative aspects of nurses, and what they are not doing, or what they do not have. When competing for status and resources, individuals fight with each other for the scarce resource, thus producing negative attitudes toward each other. Perhaps this questioning of "why" comes from a lack of assertiveness, due to years of oppression. I agree that at times nurses have articulated "Eat-or-be-eaten; it's survival." My question to this behaviour is, why do nurses feel that they are in a survival mode? What are they trying to preserve? Is it heir self-esteem? One response to nurses' behaviour toward each other included: "I don't think it's our profession, else we would be trying to support and encourage one another." In so expressing his views, this nurse blamed nurses for the lack of collegial behaviour. This attitude of looking inward to explain a lack of collegiality that exists within the profession causes a continuation of conflictual behaviours.

179

With the traditional hierarchies, staff nurses are struggling to reconcile their image and their work within a health care system in which they have little power. Staff nurses engage in behaviours consistent with the values and beliefs that has particular meaning for nursing. Most of the behaviours discussed here are associated with recognition of the culture of the profession. Staff nurses see a multitude of problems relating to patients, the system, and the profession. How they perceive and share those problems produce the interactions that occur among them. These behaviours become collegial behaviours or conflictual behaviours. As B.D. (1995) stated:

> Sometimes we have to look very hard to see our strengths rather than the problems. I would prefer friendly, compassionate support for one another so that we might emphasize our connections instead of our disconnections.

When behaviour in nursing is observed and discussed by nurses, it tends to be concentrated on the disconnections within the group; however, staff nurses want connections with their peers. Despite the interpersonal problems that occur between them, many staff nurses express the sentiments in the statement quoted above. The wish for collegial behaviour constantly challenges staff nurses, as they review the day-to-day interactions of their peers.

In this chapter I have considered behaviours relating to collegiality. In concluding, I have taken a conjectural look at some of the conditions, once removed, that seem to ensure collegial interactions. How far can we generalize from reviewing the behaviour of nurses? Behaviour patterns on units are similar when dealing with complaining, or support. We may think that nurses in psychiatry would have better communication than those in other areas. In my observations, however, their encounters are much the same as those in other areas of the hospital. Helping and caring is important to staff nurses, and when peers are in need, that behaviour comes to the forefront. When cultivated, helping peers can produce supportive, collegial behaviour that favours staff nurses. This will allow staff nurses to take more risk, to complain about each other less, and to trust each other rather, than "watching their backs."

Behaviour at the staff nurse level is related to the structure of the profession and the culture of the profession. Whatever the interaction, staff nurses deal with each other face-to-face. Events that occur in the health care system, within their profession, and in their hospitals influence matters of courtesy, and nursing collegiality. We can understand the propensity for negative behaviours to occur where stress, oppression, and powerlessness are factors within the environment. Defining these face-to-face interactions influences the attitudes that staff nurses have towards their peer group. I have attempted to show these interactions, while reviewing the questions in the survey and provide a forum for the voices of staff nurses to be heard in the explanations regarding their behaviours. Collegiality as Styles envisioned it is not part of the everyday communication at the staff nurse level, however, we witnessed an understanding of the interactions that affect staff nurses and their feeling about these interactions.

Conceptually, collegiality is more a leadership and a sexist concept. First, as discussed in chapter three, collegiality has not been discussed as behaviours that men in their professions should attain. Secondly, collegiality as described by Styles can be used to control behaviour. Thirdly, collegiality has been discussed and constructed by a small group of elites within the profession to determine what the majority "should do." The power relationships, and the bureaucratic relationships make it very unlikely that a low status group would be allowed to set the concepts of collegiality. For groups such as the nursing profession, self-disciplining depends on whether a group already has sufficient power to resist efforts by other groups to impose their discipline on them. Perhaps the leaders within the profession think they have a broader understanding of the profession and, therefore, of collegiality. It could also be that the leadership has goals for professional equality with physicians, and do poorly with nurses' daily working conditions. That is not to say that they do not write about the working conditions of the staff nurse but there is, however, a lack of effort to implement a culture that really values the work of the staff nurse. For collegiality to have meaning at the staff nurse level, there needs to be a change in attitudes, both at the leadership level, and at the level of the staff nurse.

Finally, for collegiality to exist racism and horizontal violence must be addressed within the profession, and persons who practice these behaviours need to be sanctioned, and be re-educated. Nurse leaders acknowledge the existence of rights when it comes to gender and sexism; yet, they shy away from other human rights, such as racism. They do not appear to have an investment in changing the disproportionate share of unsatisfactory roles and tasks assigned to racialised nurses; and pushing for the restructuring of nursing education to combat racism. This would require them to not merely

181

present arguments but to also push for changes to practices that would bring about racial justice, and representation. Coming together to challenge privilege, and to transform the system, would be to share in shaping the profession, providing a healthy work environment for nurses, rejecting hierarchies, and celebrating social justice, and inclusion.

Chapter Six

Understanding Issues for Advocacy

Feminists have pointed out that traditionally men have exercised power over women and in general are viewed as having less power than men in society (see Prince and Silva-Wayne 2004). An argument could have been made that when this oppressed gender had power, because of their experience, they would recognize hierarchical and abusive relationships that are harmful to women, and would be advocates for social justice within the workplace, and in society. Yet, nurse interactions have been referred to as oppressed group behaviour (Freshwater 2000)—not reacting to those oppressing them, and instead, turning on each other. To gain power and autonomy within the health care team, nursing turned to the male tradition of professionalism (Jacobs 2005). Rather than focusing on "the caring" aspect of the occupation, they promoted professionalism, and within it, collegiality.

The concept of collegiality is used within many professions to describe positive behaviours. The more frequently the concept is used within professional discourse, the more it is taken into account, and described as a professional characteristic. Often nurses who discuss conditions of nurses' work are the ones who are in positions of power, such that a concept like collegiality is constructed from the top down. At times, in order that another characteristic—the concept of professionalism—can be promoted, those constructing the concept forget, and/or ignore the experiences of frontline participants; they then start to look for behaviours that will enhance interactions amongst members.

The tension between the ideal and reality creates uneasiness in discussions about behaviours that arise out of the culture of this work environment. The ONA wants the members of their association to know that they are committed to a programme that enhances their social and economic status. For staff nurses, they know their organization acknowledges diversity, and wants to maintain mutual trust and respect. This vision can be seen in all structures of the health care system; it is putting these policies into practice that I question. The ONA, RNAO and the OHA all have policies around harassment, racism, and sexism, however, when administrations ignore these policies, they help to create a toxic work environment.

The responses from staff nurses around how they view their profes sion, and their work environment provided us the opportunity to understand issues of social justice, and how these issues relate to their everyday lives In this book, an understanding of collegiality within the nursing profession was developed through an examination of structure, culture, and behaviour The analysis pointed to how economic and social power is tied to under standings of collegiality, conflict behaviours, and inequality. By means o their experiences, we have been able to identify areas of social inequality that come about from the use and abuse of power within the profession, and in the workplace.

As with elite social organizations, and the "constellations of inter est" exhibited by corporate boards of directors, with many having ties to political parties (Carroll 2004, 5), there is an interlock that occurs in the health care system; such interlock that is very much part of the corporate sector is also part of the structures that we have examined and is part o these structures' control over work environments. In understanding the complex arrangements of the power structures, we are provided with the history of how different formulations of power and co-operation can exist they do so, even with affirmative action laws, or progressive policies within government and within the institutions.

Of central concern to this discussion is the link between the theoret- ical constructs of nursing collegiality that are prescribed by nurse leaders and the staff nurse who labels everyday behaviours that s/he encounters Professional organizations or associations have their formal culture codi- fied to a certain level that is the descriptive culture of the association tha allows the individual to follow a code of interaction, with sanctions taking place when deviations occur. Staff nurses traditionally do not have the time or the energy to challenge the assumptions made in Styles' discussion o collegiality; nor do they reflect on the method of how these concepts come to be time-honoured by the nursing profession. They are aware, however that concepts such as collegiality provide tools for those in positions o power to exercise that power within their sphere of control.

The linking of behaviours that we see between the workers and the structures of power is an important aspect in making the connection between occupational structures, and social justice. Having a voice is more than having committee membership, and involves having a vote that really counts, such that real change can occur. Staff meetings are an area where staff nurse collegiality can be observed but staff nurses complained that a

184

these meetings, many of their peers remain silent, or that they themselves do not participate. Some of the reasons they gave for these behaviours included: (1) "not being listened to;" (2) "they don't care;" (3) "they do what they want to do anyway;" or (4) "I don't care/just doing my job."

Unit rituals such as staff meetings can promote or discourage staff nurses, given that the culture has negative qualities and does not consistently allow for true collegial behaviour. If we discuss this as an issue of justice, the resource of workers' "ideas" requires treating those ideas with respect, and not leave the burden on those who already have unequal resources, to prove, or justify their value. Valuing ideas recognizes that benefits and social contributions can be made by frontline workers, rather than solely by the classic, corporate interest within the institution.

When we look at the area of professionalism in nursing, many transformations arise from elite thinking. This is not different from the notion of globalization: Who benefits from both of these changes? We know how workers are pitted against each other when global corporations are reviewed with a lack of attention to social and environmental costs (Brecher and Costello 1998). Rather than fearing globalization, social movements in civil society are coming up with strategies to confront it in a manner that addresses justice issues. Taking some direction from these groups, staff nurse groups in Canada can use advocacy to help "stir the cappuccino." The question that we must ask ourselves is—how?

Change from Within

The nursing profession is primarily made up of the staff nurse group, however, when discussing the structures of the profession, we noted that a small group within the profession set the agenda for this occupation. The large group of staff nurses, like our silent majority in society, will need to change their habits. When possible, they need to start making their views known at every level of the health care system and the profession. Rather than simply saying that they lack power, it is vital that they recognize that rules for conduct as well as the level of co-operative group work needed for their voices to be heard. Staff nurses described "in-group" and "out-group" as two types of interactional groupings within a unit. They saw those in the "in-group" doing favours for each other and doing things together, while leaving others on the outside. The "in-group" held the power and was close to the manager, while the "out-group" saw themselves as having less of everything.

A cohesive group of staff nurses can have an effect on the manager and even control her or him. It is when favouritism occurs on the part of the manager towards certain members of the group that those left out join a sub-group within the unit. Conflict arises out of the perception of who is favoured and who is on the outside. Minority nurses have reported that they have been targeted by managers and lacked support from their peers. This type of behaviour, in which one staff is pitted against another for resources within the manager's control, provides for a culture on the unit that lacks collegiality.

Some staff nurses state that they find it difficult to deal with negative personalities, and report that collegial behaviour by definition includes working together with those with whom they do not get along. Many of the nurses interviewed stated that working together was important for good patient care. Whatever the reasons for this split, how can staff nurses come to agreement when there is conflict? Reflecting on this, there is a principle common to most of us: It is wrong to harm another person. When we deprive a peer of the opportunity to participate, to speak, and to belong, this is harm at a very basic level. Power and power sharing can ensure that skills and knowledge are effectively used to create a climate of trust and equity. Thus, the presence of in-groups and out-groups point to social justice issues—resources such as promotions, conference attendance, and patient allocation are divided up to the group that is close to management, and not by merit.

Staff nurses need to judge their own behaviours regardless of the oppressive structures within the profession. Since nurses also provide newcomers with the history of the unit and the hospital, they can share policy and process knowledge. This sharing of information allows for interaction to occur and for newcomers to the unit to understand the culture of the organization. Staff nurses must function together in time of stress such as when a cardiac code is called on a unit, and nurses work together to provide care for the patient. This is a tense situation and each staff nurse must support the other for the survival of the patient. Staff nurses know their duties, but not their rights to shape policies nor for promotion, nor for racist and other oppression to be resolved within a transparent manner. Instead of working as a group, most often individuals experiencing conflict struggle on their own to cope with what is occurring. Staff nurses working as a group can empower each other and create a climate where the institutions would reflect on the consequences of their actions before enacting policies or sweeping racism under the carpet.

Gossip and complaints that are currently part of the culture of nursing decrease unit collegiality. Staff nurses, for example, are subject to "spying" by other nurses, who review their work in order to report faults to management. On the other hand, supporting each other and playing a role within the team is considered by them to be collegial and professional. Impartiality or making a newcomer welcome rather than having to prove themselves before being accepted goes beyond one's own interest "I am not paid to do this, they should have better orientation" to that of the other person who is new to the unit and needs support. Staff nurses have to look at how they divide the world into "us and them" and what this division means for collegial behaviours. The attribution of positive characteristics to oneself and one's friends and the making of comparisons to the "other" constructs interactions such that the "other" will conform to the roles and standards that is expected of them. This is a judging that prevents true group action and is a 'divide' that those in power can use to set their agenda. To bring about change from within is to first treat the view the interest of peers as equal to their own and to advocate for change in the interest of the group or public interest and not just the self.

Staff nurses, like citizens in society more generally, must looks for actions that produce more total well being for everyone affected whenever they encounter conflictual behaviours within the hospital, the profession, and in the health care system. Staff nurses are not subordinate workers but are a group of caregivers who have freely taken on an obligation to care and help others who are in need. Like environmental activists, these women and men have a responsibility to change the toxic environment of the hospitals in which they work. Rather than going to the human rights commission or the courts, changes must first be made though the development of the self and consciousness of the issues, coming together as a group with an agenda for change and advocacy for those changes. Staff nurses work hard, some on their days off at another institution. They have family obligations as well. When is their time to give to one's professional life? Perhaps that is one reason that there is a lack of movement from the bottom to change what is occurring, is the fear of set up or backlash by managers and administrators when staff nurses actively seek redress. The rest, the silent majority, come to work, do what they have to do, and go home. Becoming involved takes energy, energy they staff nurses do not have to give due to heavy work loads and constant changes that occur with the health care system and their hospitals. When something happens to an individual staff nurse it is only at this

time that they seek others such as senior peers or union stewards for infor
mation. Many do not know about their rights under the collective agreemen
and leave it to their union to fight on their behalf. If the union representa
tive is good, then the member is lucky. This lack of interest in understanding
the collective agreement and hospital policies around equity points to a lac
of motivation and perhaps their 'dis-empowered' status. If the organizatio
is not unionized, then staff nurses look to the human rights commission t
address their grievances which fall under the human rights code or they g
within the hospital to the diversity or human resource departments for hel
in dealing with the conflict that have experienced. Diversity managers an
the human resource departments report to administrators and may not b
neutral when dealing with staff and administrator conflicts. The court i
another avenue but many people are unable to afford the cost of a goo
lawyer.

Why Not the Human Rights Route?

The OHRC in their Policy and Guidelines on Racism and Racia
Discrimination (2005) states:

> Racial harassment can have a bad effect on, or
> "poison" the places where you live, work or receive services.
> Even if the harassment is not directed at you, it can still
> poison the environment for you and others. Organizations
> and institutions operating in Ontario have an obligation to
> have in place measures to prevent and respond to breaches
> of the *Code*. They have a duty to take steps to foster envi-
> ronments that are respectful of human rights. While
> on-the-job, the following types of treatment may be indica-
> tive of racial discrimination:
> * Exclusion from formal or informal networks;
> * Denial of mentoring or developmental opportunities
>   such as secondments and training which was made avail-
>   able to others;
> * Differential management practices such as excessive
>   monitoring and documentation or deviation from written
>   policies or standard practices when dealing with a
>   racialised person;

- Disproportionate blame for an incident;
- Assignment to less desirable positions or job duties;
- Treating normal differences of opinion as confrontational or insubordinate when involved with racialised persons;
- Characterizing normal communication from racialised persons as rude or aggressive;
- Penalizing a racialised person for failing to get along with someone else (*e.g.* a co-worker or manager), when one of the reasons for the tension is racially discriminatory attitudes or behaviour of the co-worker or manager.

....It has also been established that an individual's behaviour may itself be a reaction to the experience of discrimination or the existence of a poisoned environment (OHRC 2005)

The above statement by the OHRC is positive, and provides an excellent framework for comprehending racism, and racial discrimination. Appeals to the OHRC from the documentation of nurses by scholars (Hagey et al. 2005; Collins et al. 1999) shows us, however, a commission with a lack of will to change the way business occurs within the health care system. The legal framework of human rights protection allows for claims to be handled and resolved but the process is stacked in favour of the institution, and those with economic and social power (Hagey 2002). The person bringing the claim has to spend their own money, and usually does not have the resources to do so. The institution, on the other hand, has tax-appropriated dollars at its disposal to protect the institution, and in turn, the leadership against whom the complaint is made. In effect, then, the perpetrators have available the very best the legal community can offer, while the victim is left looking for the rare lawyers who work pro bono.

The workings of the Human Rights Commission, a seeming "safety net", shows the linkage of resources to power elites. Significant problems persist in the relations between "the individual" filing the complaint, and the OHRC. The Ontario government is planning to overhaul the human rights system that currently has a massive backlog of unresolved cases, as well as slashing the time it takes for a complaint to be processed within this system. Under a proposed new model in legislation to be introduced in the spring of 2006, in order to address systemic discrimination, the commission would focus on advancing human rights, and preventing discrimination

through proactive measures, such as public education, research, and monitoring.

The government would also establish an Anti-Racism Secretariat
within the Commission that would provide recommendations and advice to
the chief commissioner about research and policy to fight racism
(*Canadian Law Today* 2006). The uneven distribution of resources between
people making a claim and those against whom a complaint has been
lodged has not been addressed, nor has the way in which the OHRC has
practiced mediation between the powerful and the powerless. The implica-
tion for outcomes and the idea that the rules are applied to co-equals come
from a belief by government that both parties will be treated equally within
the process.

In analysing this new human rights process, in spite of the expectation that social justice can be realized within the Canadian social welfare
state, the individual complainant does not have the same legal powers.
Within the human rights system, inequality of economic power eliminates
the legal conditions for the end product of legal equality. Unless human
rights victims receive the same support from investigators as victims of
domestic abuse (that is, the police, and legal and therapeutic counsel), staff
nurses who use this process are faced with mediation. It is the first step
valued within the human rights system, and helps to bring the parties
together to achieve understanding. Some type of sanctions are required
when systemic racism, targeting, set-up, and backlash occur in institutions.
This would help to stop those with economic and social power from
normalizing promotion based on in-group status, horizontal violence,
racism, and aggressive discourse.

Why Not Mediation?

Mediation, a form of alternative dispute resolution, is a voluntary confidential process of discussion and direct negotiation by the parties involved in a
dispute in the presence of a trained, experienced, neutral advisor outside of
the court. Unlike judges they do not decide the case. A false premise of this
process is that the disputing parties have roughly equal bargaining power.
All individuals who file complaints with the Ontario Human Rights
Commission (ORHC) are currently offered mediation services before a
complaint is investigated. Approximately 65-70 per cent of complaints in
which mediation was attempted are successfully settled according to the

annual report of the ORHC. This number seems to suggest a positive outcome, especially when the average age of the case inventory was 11.2 months on March 31, 2005 and the total new complaints 2,339 (Ontario Human Rights Commission; Annual Report 2005). If only a small number of cases get referred to the tribunal, then mediation would be the preferred route for those who are seeking justice in terms of equality rights.

Mediation is complicated and not impartial. Under certain legal systems such as family law and human rights complaints, mediation must be resorted to by those wishing to seek redress. Those mediating must try to broker agreements. The individual such as the staff nurse who turns to the tribunal for justice now has to face those s/he is accusing of inequity as well as a mediator who has the power to decide his/her case and write a report. The mediator is not dealing with two equals but with one that has less resources than the other. Understanding this inequity would allow for mediators to acknowledge at the very beginning that the parties are not equal and that one party has institutional resources behind them while the other is paying out of pocket. The out-of-court settlement for one party, the individuals with economic and social resources can wait and do not have to settle through mediation if their agenda is not met as they have the institutional resources to provide for their legal action while the staff nurse has little or no resources and a long battle is difficult for them to sustain. Staff nurses understand compromise. Compromise is necessary for everyone to accommodate the needs for days off that each nurse requires to go to classes, keep appointments and so forth. Included in this understanding of compromise are the notions of sharing, and concern for other staff nurses. When they look for justice, however, because of what has occurred in the workplace and within their profession, compromise is more about giving up rights than bringing about understanding. Perhaps this can be a reason that the largest group of nurses, the staff nurse group, are detached from the profession and from one another. When interviewing this group of nurses, I found they felt that the legal system, because of cost, the OHRC and because of process were not worth the time, energy, and money to take on management for behaviours that were against the labour code or the ORHC code. In terms of turning to the union, they felt they had a weak union and that administration prolonged the process and the union could not do anything to stop this type of behaviour. "What's the use!" was a common phrase, with an indication that mediation worked in favour of the administration.

Bringing two unequal groups together so that the parties can move beyond hostility, suspicion, and avoidance to address the dispute that divides them is like asking an abused wife to meet her husband and address why he is beating her; legal action is clearly the more appropriate course with restraining orders for the husband. When racism or sexism has been the root cause of a problem, a mediator might de-emphasize these issues in order to avoid inflaming hostility and so reach an agreement more efficiently. This is seeking to help both parties but is also enabling the perpetrator, rather than empowering the one who has experienced the abuse. The mediator's objective is to promote greater understanding, and bring about a new relationship.

What about protecting the rights of those who do not have social and economic power? Why is it that in the mediating process individuals such as a staff nurse have to "give up" their rights to accommodate the administrators, who have both social and economic power? Seeking to accommodate when it comes to systemic racism, bullying, harassment, violence, and other oppressions can be harmful, as we are trying to justify a behaviour, and not deal with the harm done by the behaviour.

As we have seen, nurses have reported to the researcher that they have been abused and harassed by peers, physicians, other hospital employees, patients, and visitors; and this is especially true for minority nurses. The reinforcing patterns of the workplace discourage staff nurses from reporting abuse, to tolerate abuse from physicians, and to tolerate abuse from patients. Coupled with this is the fact that there is insufficient follow-through on harassment and racism policies by that administration. Several respondents expressed the belief that the administration "does not view this as an important" issue and that "nothing will be done." In interviews staff nurses told me that if senior managers who "sit in offices" could relate differently with frontline staff, and if administrators had "face-to-face" interactions, either individually, or at the group level, it would be encouraging to staff, and would raise their morale. This contact could lead to a climate that encourages staff to ask questions, and to propose recommendations for change. The nurses recognise that trust and respect comes from a nurtured relationship, and a safe environment for open communication.

The professional structure of nursing has also not adopted an outspoken role in promoting racialised minority views and concerns. In my observation, they come to policies and concerns about nursing from the dominant group's viewpoint. When discussing the structures of the profession racialised nurses were excluded by the MoH in discussions around the future of the profession as many do not belong to senior management and are not in positions of power. We can view this as systemic behaviours of harassment and racism. When we look at senior administration within the health care system, we see white privilege. As with the practice of anti-racist advocates, staff nurses need to organize and monitor complaints. Their union and professional association like most institutions in society have deep-rooted attitudes about nursing, which arises from racial-group membership. Racism is embedded in the dominant culture and is deep-rooted in our institutions in a way that is pervasive, often invisible, and tolerated.

Mediation in such cases is inadequate, and allows for white privilege to continue. Until we have a workplace and professional structures reflecting Canada's racial and ethnic diversity, mediation around issues such as racism, and other oppressions mentioned above, must be within an anti-racism praxis. Such action is oppositional to white hegemony and the attending social, economic, and political interests; it is also oppositional to the power and privilege that is invisible to those who possess it. This is also about a form of social action that is transforming, even if it means making one party uncomfortable during the implementation of the reforms. Mediation being a process that is about bringing parties together does not work in the best interest of those bringing complaints that fall under the ORHC.

Why Advocacy?

Social distance between staff nurses needs to be eliminated. Regrettably, the individual staff nurse tends to assume that she or he cannot change the culture of nursing within the hospital or the profession. Political action is necessary in order for the staff nurse to influence the culture of nursing, and for political action to occur, individual staff nurses must unify and strive for collective improvements. Only group unity can possibly lead to empowerment and a true collegial culture. Unless staff nurses undertake actions to promote their needs and to promote critical awareness in the public at large around shortages within the health care system, the bureaucratic organizational structures and its hierarchy place staff nurses in a subordinate position.

193

Powerlessness in concert with a professional culture that produces a breakdown in solidarity and therefore collegiality leads to individuals feeling isolated. Collegiality seems like a flexible concept when in action in the everyday delivery of patient care. When an attack comes from the outside, members pull together, and solidarity increases, which brings about an increase in collegial behaviours.

Issues of social justice, including the injustices that staff nurses' experience in the workplace and in the profession, must include analysis of aggressions and inequities in representations to government and the community. We live in a very complex and diverse society that contains many voices. ONA and the RNAO must include voices 'from the margins' on an ongoing basis, enabling them to bring their issues to 'the centre'. For change to occur, rather than focusing on the dysfunctional nurse-nurse behaviours, the focus of the message, and the use of resources in a purposeful, directed manner, will not only empower the nurse but will also improve nursing care.

Although the current environment in the health care system pits nurse against nurse, when negative behaviours towards them occurs, the staff nurse group has at least three choices: they can resist, accommodate, or consent to what is happening. Resisting can take the form of advocacy, control of their union, and control of their profession. As they are the largest group in nursing, staff nurses, like the silent majority are responsible for their leadership due to their lack of participation at the organization level and in voting. Staff nurses must act together and have strategies to dissuade behaviours that would prevent the development of a climate of collegiality. They are members of the nursing community, and until they view it as their responsibility to bring about shared equity, change will not occur.

As noted earlier, nursing is not a culture where staff nurses are called upon to support ideas, and where they are included in the initiation of change. To involve themselves with change, and interact with their peers within the hospital, would mean that staff nurses would have to go beyond their unit boundaries. For this to occur, units need to be linked with each other to provide information as to what is going on within each unit, and what they know is happening within the hospital. At the hospital level, there is currently a shift from interaction between a small number of staff nurses within a specific unit, to the large group of staff nurses working within a hospital. Although hospitals are bureaucratic, having a voice means communication in the making of rules. Those nurses involved in committees provide a voice for their colleagues, and their actions can be viewed as advocating for the goals of the entire group. Their identity is not of the self but as a staff nurse speaking on behalf of her or his peers.

Communication is then another behaviour that is needed by staff nurses in order to keep those who are not involved informed as to what is happening at the hospital and professional levels. If this was to occur, alienation within the profession would decrease, and perhaps collegiality would increase for the staff nurse at the professional level. Involvement in the processes of change and of running the hospital by those who have been excluded leads to ownership not only of the processes but to institutional change.

The elites within the health system, just like the elites within society, control and direct the polity to protect their interest and not the benefit of the staff nurses. The worth of the staff nurse, like the worth of other workers, is set by others. It is therefore in the best interest of the staff nurse group to set standards and that their role within the hospital and the health care system is treated with respect. Advocacy involves making those around you aware of the issues that need attention and change. Educating them of the facts and building a bridge in the minds of those you need to impact becomes a way of taking control of the change agenda. Part of the struggle to get the message out is related to both economic and social power.

Teaching Advocacy

Advocacy is a set of actions that can set in motion social change. Industry and professional organizations as well as non-governmental organizations use different approaches to advocate their positions. Advocacy can take time, energy, and other resources. The questions most often asked are, "How do I advocate?" and "Who will listen to me?" The two questions do not have direct answers, however, in order to achieve some level of success we need to build bridges with other like-minded individuals as well as individuals in positions of power, especially within government and business. Our focus is to make them aware of our concerns regarding social conditions, policies, and actions that are harmful to the citizenship in general. We may want to make them mindful of the difference between merely understanding discrimination and changing the environment that supports these injustices. In the discussion of education, health and social service we have separate silos which allows for the status quo to exist. It is in the intersection of race, class, and gender and the integration of different institutions that will allow for an alteration of the structures that support current toxic environments and will help produce healthy social relations for the collective. It is through community interaction and advocacy that social relations can be addressed and changed.

Tactics for Increasing Awareness

- Coordinate effort between other individuals who want change.
- Coordinate efforts between organizations.
- Contact business leaders in your area who may wish to support the issue.
- Drop off relevant literature at your MPP's office with your name and telephone number.
- Meet with your local MP/MPP.
- Obtain a commitment from the MP/MPP to take the message to the Minister.
- Follow-up with local MPP.
- Local action includes letters and petitions to your MPP.
- Call the Premier's office and Minister's office to express your views.
- Local action with media includes monitoring coverage, letters to the editor, and contacting friendly reporters with key messages.
- Letters to the editor in order to continue to generate awareness.
- Start a petition/sign a petition; take it to your local MP/MPP and ask him or her to deliver it to the Minister.

Your Key Messages: Why are They Important?

Whenever you converse with business leaders, leaders or members of other organizations, or your political leaders, you must have a message that is consistent and prepared.

Key messages are the issues that you and your group have put together that you wish to get across. Use research and published articles to

196

create your Key Messages that you wish to present when advocating for social change. It does not matter if the change is in the area of health, gender or race discrimination. More than five Key Messages are difficult to absorb, so do not exceed this total, and keep these key aspects of your communication as uncomplicated as possible. This is also important when writing to the editor.

- *Research is key.* Remember that you are trying to distinguish your organization and your issue from many other very worthwhile issues. Prepare yourself for the style as well as the substance of the meeting. Knowing your audience, how they operate, and what they need and want from groups like yours can make a huge difference. The deeper the impression you make, the better the odds that your cause will be recognized by the MP/MPP and as such you will be able to influence his or her actions.
- *A good case contains a clear and simple statement of your issue.* It is well researched, competently analysed, and focused on a clear set of issues. It presents a straightforward conclusion and where necessary offers realistic alternatives.
- *Tell part of your case as a teacher would.* Polish your stories to make a point. Personalize them so the person you are speaking to (MP/MPP) has a powerful tool to take on to other audiences; personal cases can have more of an affect than abstractions. MPs/MPPs want the support of others in order that they are not in the forefront for change by themselves.
- *A persuasive case is simply a good case that has been tailored for specific use in the public arena.* Most public groups stop with a good case. What this type of case most often fails to do is convey the emotional importance of the issue—either your sense of commitment or its importance to the MP/MPP. You must keep in mind the policy framework in which government operates and it is in this area that you must make a tailored case that is persuasive for not only the individual you are speaking or writing to but also in such a way that she or he can take your materials to their caucus and the community at large.

There is a difference between a face-to-face meeting and writing a letter, however, in both communications remember to prepare, prepare, prepare.

Steps to a Successful Meeting with an MP/MPP

1. Prepare. Prepare. Prepare. Set your objectives and develop your strategy and communications plan before you make any phone calls. Key messages are a must.

2. Research your local MPP's views on what you are presenting. Does he or she have any personal experiences in the area? When meeting with local business or other organizations, research their views and their structures. Can you find common ground for shared concerns, or a common interest?

3. Decide with whom you want to meet. In some cases, the more influential the MP/MPP (i.e., a cabinet minister), the more difficult it will be to schedule a meeting. An initial meeting with a staff person may be a worthwhile first step, however, indicate your desire to meet with the MP/MPP in the future. This also applies to business leaders.

4. Think about timing. *Fridays* are usually constituency days and a good meeting day. In addition, when the legislature is not sitting, MP/MPPs are often in their constituency office much of the time.

5. Send a letter (by fax, where possible) requesting an opportunity to meet. Follow up by phone with the staff and ask for a commitment for the meeting date and time. Continue to call once every week until a meeting is scheduled. Remember to ask how long you have with the MP/MPP. If the allotted time is insufficient, ask for more. Usually you may only get 15 minutes and need to prepare for getting your message across within this time frame.

6. Ask appropriate people to accompany you. Prepare them ahead of time with objectives and key messages. Agree beforehand who will address what issues.

7. Prepare an information package to be sent one week prior to your meeting. Ask the individual to review material before the meeting. Include information on the provincial and local organization, relevant statistics, information on your current initiatives, any national or provincial papers, policies, or motions supporting your issue. The meeting will be more productive if both groups are prepared. Include a meeting agenda in the package.

8. Prior to the meeting, decide what types of information and commitments you want to have when you leave the meeting. Be specific. Ask for a specific reply or action by a specific date. There is a difference between meeting with business leaders and leaders of other organizations and when you meet with politicians. With the former, you need to have issues that they see as important for either their membership or their consumers. With politicians, they are responsible to their constituency.

9. When meeting with a politician, you may need to have a second meeting before you get any commitments. *Be persistent.* Be prepared with an action that you can suggest to a very sympathetic MP/MPP.

10. Begin the meeting by stating why you requested the meeting and what you hope to accomplish. If possible, use handouts to help communicate your information. Keep it simple. Remember that these individuals are not specialists on your issue. Keep it relatively brief—the more influential MP/MPPs have the greatest time pressures and will appreciate a succinct persuasive presentation.

11. Use references from the research you have done on their office regarding their position of the issue. Offer ways in which the MP/MPP's office can benefit from supporting your organization or your issue. For example, your organization could include their names in their newsletter, invite them to speak at monthly meetings, or include them in community awareness days. Remember that MP/MPPs are elected and their goal is to stay in that

position by being well known, well liked, and active in their community.

12. End the meeting by asking for a commitment to respond by a specific date or schedule another meeting to discuss next steps and the commitment you are looking for. Once again, be specific.
13. Write a follow-up letter outlining the issues discussed and next steps for both groups (if applicable). Send the letter to the MP/MPP's office within five business days of the meeting and copy all people in attendance.
14. Contact organizations that are supportive to your objectives with the results of your efforts!

Ten Steps to a Successful Letter Writing Campaign

1. Set your objective for the letter writing campaign—what outcome do you want? To change or influence policy?
2. Develop key messages to be included in the letters. The key messages should reflect the focus and objective of the campaign.
3. *Do not use form letters.* Politicians and bureaucrats discount these letters because they appear too staged. Varying each letter allows for the personal importance and emotion of the issue to be communicated. Provide participants in the letter writing campaign with key messages, names, and addresses so they can create their own letter.
4. Ask for a specific action in the letters. For example, ask MP/MPPs to express their support for your issue or cause publicly, and to seek the support of their colleagues in caucus.
5. Back up your request with statistics and research to demonstrate the importance of the issue. Don't be afraid to use personal examples. This will ensure the MP/MPP understands your side of the issue.
6. Provide participants in the letter writing campaign with a deadline for their letters. Ask them to report back when the letter is complete.

7. Send the letters to the MPP's constituency address and make sure all the letters are personalized. Send copies of the letters to the Minister and the Premier.

8. Schedule the letter-writing campaign for greatest affect. A particularly good time is 6-12 months before an election, however it can be anytime. The timing can also reflect local events.

9. Follow up the letters with phone calls to recipients to ensure the letters were received, to increase the awareness of the issues and to stress the need for action.

10. Ask for a formal response from the MP/MPP. Report back to the participants on the number and quality of the responses. Always make sure to send a thank-you letter to the MP/MPP. Your advocacy is not just for your benefit, it is because it will make a difference for a group. The MP/MPP knows this and wants to be part of the big picture. Time is important; acknowledge the MP/MPP for spending time on the important issues you presented.

Advocacy is not limited to the few samples provided in this chapter. The purpose of advocacy is to promote an understanding of the actions needed if we want action to occur. In addition, it takes energy and time from our busy lives to advocate for others and ourselves. The above ideas when implemented indicate that individuals and members of organizations have valuable expertise and can give legitimacy when they contact people in positions of power. Critical decisions are made within government without the input or the knowledge of the citizens until it is too late for action. We need to ensure we have information about the changes that are occurring around us via the media or through other sources. The reader needs to move from understanding to tackling the problems that face us in society. Reform can only occur when we take action. Social change and advocacy go hand in hand. The more voices heard by those in power, the less likely they will act on issues that are not in the best interest of women and other minorities within our society.

Advocacy does not exist in a vacuum. There are contexts, arguments, and issues that are part of a wider debate. Entering into this debate takes energy. Rather than polarization, advocacy relates to the power structures and tries to weaken agendas that do not address the needs of the group by expressing the realities of those seeking change. New perspectives rooted in the experiences of those at the margins advocate for different or new rights and rules. To organize and raise awareness is to build co-operation among members who once were silent. The ability for staff nurses, like citizens in society more generally, to affect the upward levelling of the conditions of those at the bottom can be viewed as a shift from the margins to the centre.

Empowerment can only come from action. This construction of collegiality from the staff nurse group is about actions that occur and actions that need to occur. Staff nurses, who are mostly women, must understand the struggle and the consciousness of their position within the system, must construct their vision of the nursing profession, and not leave it to the elites within the profession. After all, there are far more staff nurses than management staff, and other staff within the professional hierarchy. Until staff nurses view their numbers in terms of power and understand social justice, the small yet powerful group of females in nursing will continue to construct and promote their view of the profession and of collegiality, just as the elites in society who make laws which enhance their lives.

Advocacy for Social Justice Issues

An examination of behaviours in the workplace provides a window for the understanding of the culture that allows such behaviours to exist or take place. This culture is produced by structures with systemic issues that are in need of changing, and to just address the behaviour of staff nurses and try to find reasons for it will not address the systemic issues. When behaviours between staff nurses and administrators occur, some look to mediation, diversity officers, and OHRC processes. There is a place for these interventions, however, past experience shows us that it not only has taken time but also that the outcomes have not moved the structures in a new direction; they have paid lip service to change but have continued to sidestep the problems. Those who have been distressed have called others like themselves for support. With a lack of funds and many times with the lack of union support, they give up and withdraw. In my study, the expression of the feeling that "things will not change" by nurses was common. Some in leadership positions think that they can use mediation to have a win-win situation where those with economic and social power will feel included and not become hostile to the changes that are needed within the profession. I find this thinking to be limiting, as those in power do not want to change and have to be told that their behaviours are unacceptable. Their actions must be sanctioned rather than mediated. If we need to change the structures where oppression occurs, there must be an overall shift—instead of depending on mediation and human rights commissions, staff nurses, student nurses, and racialised managers and professors in nursing, like the citizens in our society more generally, need to view their role in society as an advocate for themselves and others. Through the conception of advocacy, the staff nurse constructs the message and looks for partners to change professional and work structures so that equity and accountability is practiced. These voluntary actions have power, and a large group empowering themselves changes their social position as the least important to one whose voice becomes acknowledged by the economic and social elites. Once those in power know that their actions will set into motion protest in the form of advocacy by a large group, the full implications of making decisions for the benefit of all parties involved can become the new norm. The white female managers and professors may think they are progressive, but their actions when dealing with others, as described in this book, shows us that they do not walk the talk. Stirring the coffee means they will have to give up control and allow other competent racialised nurses to take roles of leadership. Up until the present time, this is not occurring, and therefore advocacy is needed to change how this profession is managed and controlled. If we leave it to those in power to provide change on our behalf, the four structures named in this book will continue to be white at the top.

Advocacy is not censoring or shaming, but rather ensuring that rights and rules are applied and that some are not treated with privilege while others are marginalized. The dominant narratives of social and economic values can and must include the narratives of the marginalized, the frontline workers. Employment structures at every stage become a site of struggle when inclusion is not viewed as an economic advantage. Group advocacy can help change the low status of frontline workers and their position in the workplace and within their professions. The administrative class and the political class, when provided with key messages, will learn that there are benefits from the feedback when change needs to occur. Changing structures where those in power are comfortable takes energy. There will be resistance even if it is passive in nature. Advocacy about the need for corporate responsibility to open doors to staff so that they participate at every level of the organization means that staff must be vigilant to all memos and new directions.

Using the strategies outlined above, nurses can come together and present their message. An example of nursing advocacy can be observed in the actions of an organization, The Centre for Equity in Health and Society (CEHS), which is a non-profit organization in Ontario. Their Board of Directors is made up of representatives from the following supporting organizations: The Barbados Nurses Association of Canada (Toronto Chapter), Chinese Canadian Nurses Association (CCNA), Coalition of Black Trade Unionists, Ontario Chapter (CBTU), The Filipino Nurse Association, The Grenada Nurses Association, Korean Nurses Association of Ontario (KNAO), Rainbow Health Network (RHN), The South Asian Nurses Association of Canada, University Hospital of the West Indies Graduate Nurses' Association (UHWIGNA), Urban Alliance on Race Relations (UARR), Eritrean Canadian Nurses Association in Ontario CEHS is calling for dialogues on anti-racism throughout the Canadian nursing profession to create effective accountability policies that will ensure that the work environment for nurses, and, therefore, for patients, is caring rather than poisoned. Such policies, as they pertain to systemic racism in nursing, would govern local, provincial, and national programs and practices. They would ensure safety for racialised nurses; especially during periods of under funding for nursing that involve restructuring and down-sizing.

CEHS has documented millions of health care dollars being spent on grievances and complaints charging employers with discrimination or harassment. Their research reported racial tension, poor handling of disputes and a reduction in diversity during times of under-funding and down sizing, (Hagey, Lum, MacKay, Turrittin and Brody 2001). The research program findings at the CEHS strongly supported the need for the development and implementation of an accountability tool for use in nursing employment and through formal channels asked to dialogue with Canadian nurse leaders, Joint Provincial Nursing Committee, on this agenda. Nursing leaders do not lend their support for such action, and remain silent on many of these issues; however, staff nurses and racialised nurses contact the CEHS for advice and help. ONA Local 097 approached CEHS for advice when they experienced ONA Central's unjust conclusions Using advocacy, CEHS through letter writing, meeting with MPPs and other state holders explained how duly elected racialised nurses were removed by their union, the ONA where there was no proof of either financial mismanagement or election irregularities by the Local. In their advocacy for these nurses CEHS points to racially based conflict as the basis of the crisis and urges MPPs and other organizations to help the nurses and support the Ontario Human Rights Commission to undertake an investigation of systemic discrimination at ONA. This type of collective action informs government and representatives of the issues and it lends support to those who are experiencing racially based actions.

What is occurring relates not just to their legal rights but also to their moral rights. By decertifying this Local, they tainted the character of the Local leaders and used their dues to take them to court. There is a moral argument attached to the legal rights of these nurses. The four racialised nurses who were fighting for their rights by contacting the CEHS, now have a larger group of concerned individuals and organizations speaking out on their behalf. Those experiencing injustice expect that the problems that have been created will be addressed through several strategies. The use of representation at the Ontario Labour Relation Board, the filing of complaints with the Ontario Human Rights Commission and requesting CEHS to help inform those in government of an important issues relating to the nursing profession in Toronto. All this comes at a time when governments are trying to keep nurses in the profession due to the shortage of nurses in Canada (A Report on The Nursing Strategy for Canada 2003). In reviewing their action CEHS is proactive by identifying the issues relating to racism and tries problem solving rather than blaming. From this perspective it is the solution to the problem that is being advocated as well CEHS though advocacy is stating that it is unjust to violate racialised nurses' legal and moral rights.

Changing attitudes around sexism, racism, and other oppressions requires sustained advocacy as well as the use of the legal and human rights system when necessary. The human rights system alone does not work. Social justice comes from ideas, reason, and arguments about basic moral questions. These questions arise in the context of governments and civil society. Therefore, the nature of inequity and its practiced must be made public. For many, when they are treated in an unjust manner, no one hears about the behaviours, however, advocacy groups can make known that which has remained silent.

The focal point for advocacy is about social justice for those who cannot speak for themselves. Injustice is structured, institutionalized and systemic. The formation of collective action by those who believe in social justice within the nursing profession depends on potential recruits and the energy they bring to promote equity. Like the environment movement, staff

205

nurses can promote the rights of nurses who have been excluded from th
health system's strategic decision-making. As well, their membershij
includes racialised nurses who need their white peers. They can use grouj
strength to advocate for a collegial work environment using collectiv
action such as advocacy. The feature of advocacy is an attempt to maximiz
the message of all the individuals involved in sending it. Governmen
responds to groups that lobby and petition their MPs\MPPs. Acting alon
is hard but acting within a group can help change institutionalized oppres
sion. Inside hospitals, staff nurses will continue to feel the pressure o
heavy workloads, the change in government policies and funding, the lacl
of real input into hospital policies that influences their work and the issue
of gender, race, class and entrenched hierarchies of hospital life. Th
culture where this occurs provides answers to the question of collegiality i
nursing. The information provided for this book points to structural occu
pational injustice and how the staff nurse group can use advocacy to hel
change their work environment.

Conclusion

Women in Canada are aware that gender-neutral treatment of economic
social and cultural rights has not advanced women's equality in the paic
labour force. Women are still performing the majority of the work in the
'caring' occupations and this 'women's work' is usually lower paid thar
'men's work'. I have tried to look into nursing, a profession dominated b
women and one of the 'caring' occupations to interpret the behaviours tha
women in power act in their own interest and control the agenda that advan
tage the dominant group. This profession within the health care system, anc
like other systems in society, it is deeply structured around hierarchies—
these hierarchies are based on interlocking influences of race, ethnicity
class, and gender. Given the barriers that block full economic participatior
for some classes of nurses within the nursing profession I looked at stan
dards pertaining to professionalism and collegial behaviour and found tha
the largest group of nurses were dissatisfied with the leadership, thei
concerns not viewed as important and reported a toxic work environment
The lack of accountability needs to be addressed by the CNO, OHA and the
MoH.

In Ontario, the study of racism within nursing has been spearec
headed by racialised scholars. Research in the area of racism in nursing

although limited, is systematic and untangles the complexities to help solve particular problems within the profession and work environment. In my discussions, I note the distribution of administrative employment opportunities across all four structures discussed in this book is white on the top. This information comes from local knowledge provided by staff nurses as well as the few racialised managers and academics. We can check university, hospital and professional organization website information regarding the individuals in leadership positions and the reader will find that it is mostly white at the top. The issues that were explored in this book are a step in the journey to stir the cappuccino—white on top, brown on the bottom.

Throughout this book, I also discussed how limited staff nurses felt within the structures of their profession and within the hospital. In 2006 nurses in discussions with me report that there is still lack or no support for staff, lack of input from management 'other than point finger of blame. DB continued to state that she had 'sleep disturbance, and feel I have no choice but to resign. I don't want to work for an organisation that blatantly does not care for their staff' (April 2006). It would appear that since 1994 very little has changed for front line staff nurses. As a class of nurses they find themselves outside the discussion making structure of the profession, the work environment and the health care system. Substantial organisation and investment is needed to include this group of workers when dealing with service improvements, reorganization and risk management strategies. Labour participation is an important area for advocacy. Staff nurse need to advocate for the right to participate and the right to fair treatment. When the individual joins with others, this power multiplies. To understand this is to understand advocacy and to understand why this tool is important in the area of social and economic justice. Using advocacy as a tool I sought to provide one type of solution to help in breaking down barriers to full participation, both in our work lives and in civil society. Out of the 86,168 nurses working in Ontario, there are 69,943 who are in direct care (CNO Statistical Report 2004). If this large group of nurses do not have a voice in current changes that are occurring within the health care system, and within their own profession, we must ask the question of morale within the system. It is important too to question the 'buy-in' by front line workers to the changes that are taking place, and to encourage their allegiance to the profession.

What is occurring in hospitals cuts across race, ethnicity, and class, and is fuelled through the network of relationships that currently exists for the ruling class within this profession. Those staff nurses chosen to participate within 'the network' are those who are groomed for the inner circle within the nursing profession. It is not that staff nurses or visible minority nurses do not know how to network; the issue is about how they are allowed to participate within "the network", and whether they are welcomed as equals to participate within the power structure. The findings point to an inner group that has constructed control over decision-making and has expectations of entitlement. The process of giving voice to oppression and domination in the legal language of social and economic rights would foster public discussions about the need for equality in concrete terms. That kind of action would prevent the powerful from evading their social responsibility, and will make them walk the talk. In addition, those individuals who are experiencing oppression and domination must learn to push back and take control of their agenda. Staff nurses can change their profession and the workplace—they need to stir this cappuccino.

Canada, in our discussions is viewed as a democratic country that promotes human rights in policies and through Acts of government. Social justice with its history in religion and philosophy is difficult to define but is viewed as part of our social fabric. The area of social and economic justice that has many dimensions provided a springboard to pursue non-supportive behaviours and injustices within occupational structures. Yet those seeking equality through the OHRC find themselves battling those in power and not getting the promised results.

Today, economic, social and cultural rights are especially relevant to human rights dialogue. While the International Covenant on Economic Social and Cultural Rights *(UN Fact Sheet No. 16, 1991)* sets out an international framework for protection of these rights, there are few mechanisms for enforcement. Evidence provided by staff nurses about their profession and their work environment, raised questions regarding the appropriate processes for hiring, promotion, and wage distribution. Economic justice helps us focus on the concerns of social justice, so that equal opportunity and the end of overt discrimination in hiring practices are important parts of the discourse that needs to take place. This will ensure representation and promote multiculturalism but it is not followed within all workplace environments.

The voices of staff nurses and racialised nurses described a line separating the leaders from them, and of inequity in hiring and promotions. These nurse leaders work on agendas that are important to them, rather than getting true input from staff nurses. Power and knowledge are intertwined

208

and so nurse leaders use resources to mobilize policy debates. This approach limits the majority of nurses from participating in the change process as they lack resources and information about the process. This allows the power elites to advocate on most knowledge issues, curriculum, on changes to the health system, best practices, cultural competencies and the role of nurses within the health care system. Perhaps this may be part of the reason for nurses leaving the profession, and also for women seeking other occupations, as they no longer have to work in a pink ghetto (Jacobs 2006). If the profession does not meet the needs of the staff nurse group or comprehends their work and what is important to them, then it will not attract or retain its membership.

Feminist scholars engaged with the questions relating to women's work need to provide a strong and articulate critique of their elite sisters within the profession of nursing and must ask the trough questions regarding racism and the nature of equality within the profession and not just point to government cut backs, physicians and patriarchy. We have spent tax dollars to research nursing work life without discussing issues relating to the oppressive behaviours and lack of accountability from nurse leaders.

Most of the regulations for professions and trades fall under provincial jurisdiction that has transferred the ability to self regulate independent of the government. When authority is diversified then no one becomes accountable for racist and other oppressive behaviours that occur within the profession. The Charter creates the illusion of social change and supports a rights discourse. As the state became more involved in justice through the legal and human rights system, the state has not viewed responsibility as part of its role. The process of balancing professional autonomy and social change distorts the equality debate and helps governments evade social responsibility. Leaving it to the administrators and professional organizations to provide safeguards and policies shows how Canada values social and economic justice in the work place. A government has a duty to take appropriate legislative, administrative, budgetary, judicial and other measures to fulfil these rights and not leave it to professional and administrative elites to administer and safeguard minority rights. Social exclusion will occur when structural process allow for inequalities that arise out of oppression related to race, class, gender, disability, sexual orientation, immigrant status and religion to exist within the work and professional environments and when the government abdicates its responsibility.

Finally, questions have been raised around occupational structures and the challenges that racialised nurses and workers at the staff level experience. The OHRC acknowledges that racial discrimination also occurs in significant measure on a systemic or institutional level (2005) yet to date has not been proactive within the nursing profession. The idea that social and economic advantage is related to equity shifts the attention from the individual to those in power. Equity as discussed in this book is a process with policies in place but practices and barriers that allow for injustices continue to exist. We cannot wait for policymakers in the health system to change structural barriers for equal participation to occur.

Of central importance is the idea of breaking down barriers, and creating partnerships with progressive leaders, in order that subordinated groups can work with them on problems of exclusion. Lethargy, defeat, and feeling tired will allow for economic and social justice in the workplace to remain elusive. Building coalitions and framing the discussion takes energy but energy is generated when we support each other, and enlist progressive leaders to the cause.

The analysis regarding exclusion directs the reader to avoid old ways of dealing with those in power, and instead, to invent new ways of responding to structural oppression, and workers' cynicism. While my hope is that the learner will be inspired to engage in changing the system, I do not seek to discourage them; rather, I would wish that they be aware of the political dynamics that shape this struggle. Even those who believe in an ideal world in which all citizens are able to maximize their potential will consider the political and cultural realties, and evaluate the actions provided in this book. The many voices that spoke about injustices that exist in the workplace suggest that social and economic justice is a work in progress, and that a different approach is needed. It will be interesting to see how the various levels of governments respond to these injustices, and what they do to enforce the human rights code. It is clear that occupational structures are one of the main paths to achieving a just society. Although this book focuses on the quality of the working lives of individuals, it is the reality of occupational structures that is the main concern. For in order to move towards equality and social justice, occupational structures and workplace environments must be changed and challenged on all fronts.

References

A Report on The Nursing Strategy for Canada. 2003. Advisory Committee Health Delivery and Human Resources. Health Canada. Ottawa, Ontario http//www.hc-sc.gc.ca/english/nursing.

A Commitment to Nursing Leadership, Organization, and Policy Theme. 2005. A report prepared to highlight the Canadian Health Services Research Foundation's commitment to nursing. Ottawa, Ontario www.chsrf.ca.

Armstrong, Bromley L. 2000. *Bromley: Tireless Champion for Just Causes.* Ontario: Vitabu Publishing.

Armstrong, P. and Armstrong, H. 1990. *Theorizing Women's Work.* Toronto: Garamond Press.

Armstrong, P., Choiniere. J., and Day, E. 1993. *Vital Signs: Nursing in Transition.* Toronto: Garamond.

Armstrong, P., and Armstrong, H. 1996. *Wasting Away: The Undermining of Canadian Health Care.* Ontario: Oxford University Press.

Ashley, J. A. 1976. *Hospitals, paternalism, and the role of the nurse.* New York: Teachers College Press. Columbia University.

Balsmeyer, B., Haubrich, K., and Quinn, C. 1996. "Defining Collegiality within the Academic Setting" *Journal of Nursing Education.* Vol. 35(6): 264-267.

Battiste, Marie. 2005. "You Can't Be the Global Doctor If You're the Colonial Disease". In Tripp, Peggy and Muzzin, Linda. (Ed) *Teaching as Activism: Equity meets Environmentalism.* Montreal & Kingston. McGill-Queen's University Press.

Baumann, A., and O'Brien-Pallas, L. 1993. "Nurses' Worklife: Researching the Quality" *The Canadian Nurse.* Vol. 89(1): 40-41.

Baumgart, A., and Larsen, J. 1988. "Overview: Nursing practice in Canada". In A. Baumgart and J. Larson (Eds). *Canadian nursing faces the future: Development and Change.* Toronto: C.V. Mosby.

Beach, M.C. and Price, E. G. 2005. "Cultural competence: A systematic review of health care provider educational interventions". *Medical Care.* Vol. 43(4) April.

Berdahl, Jennifer L. and Moore, Celia. 2006. "Workplace Harassment: Double Jeopardy for Minority Women". *Journal of Applied Psychology.* Vol. 91(2): 426–436.

211

Benner, P. 1982. "From Novice to Expert" *American Journal of Nursing*. March. 402-407.

Benner, P. 1984. *From Novice to Expert*. Addison: Wesley Publishing Company Inc.

Bess, J. L. 1988. *Collegiality and Bureaucracy in Modern University*. New York: Teachers College Press.

Bingham, S. 1979. *Ministering Angles*. New Jersey: Medical Economics Co. Book Division.

Boykin, A. 1995. *Power, Politics and Public Policy: A matter of caring*. New York: National League for Nursing Press.

Boyle, K. 1984. "Power in nursing: A Collaborative approach". *Nursing Outlook*. Vol. 32(3): 164-167.

Brecher, J. and Costello, T. 1998. *Global Village or Global Pillage* (2ed). South End Press. Cambridge, Massachusetts.

"Building on Values: The Future of Health Care in Canada". 2002. Government of Canada Commission Report. Chair: Roy Romanow.

Bullough, B., and Bullough, V. 1994. *Nursing Issues: for the Nineties and Beyond*. New York: Spring Publishing Company.

Byer, J. E., and Marshall, J. 1981. "The interpersonal dimension of collegiality" *Nursing Outlook*. Vol. 29(11): 662-665.

Byrne, C. 1988. "Thousand of Nurses are expected to quit over work conditions". *The Globe and Mail*. April 25. A2.

Calliste, A. 1996. Antiracism organizing and resistance in nursing: African Canadian women. *The Canadian Review of Sociology & Anthropology*. Vol. 33(3): 361-369.

_____ 2000. "Resisting professional exclusion and marginality in nursing: Women of colour in Ontario". In Kalbach, M. & Kalbach, W. (Eds), *Perspectives on ethnicity in Canada*, pp. 303-28. Toronto: Harcourt.

_____ 2000a. "Nurses and porters: Racism, sexism and resistance in segmented labour markets". In Calliste, A. & Sefa Dei, G. J. (Eds). *Anti-racist feminism: Critical race and gender studies*, pp.143-164. Halifax, NS, Canada: Fernwood.

Campbell, M. 1988. "Management as Ruling: A Class Phenomenon in Nursing". *Studies in Political Economy*. Autumn, 27.

Canadian Law Today. 2006. http://www.employmentlawtoday.com/login Area/guestview.asp?articleid=937.

Canadian Multiculturalism Act. 1988, c. 31, assented to 21st July, 1988 *An Act for the preservation and enhancement of multiculturalism in Canada* http://www.pch.gc.ca/progs/multi/policy/act_e.cfm.

Carlisle, D. 1990. "Trying to Open Doors: Racism in Nursing" *Nursing Times.* (May 2) Vol. 86(18): 42-43.

Carroll, William, K. 2004. *Corporate Power in a Globalizing World: A Study in Elite Social Organization.* Ontario: Oxford University Press.

CBC News online. 2004. "Taking the pulse of nurses". September 7, 2004.

CBC News online. 2006. "Dying for a job: Health-care workers beware". April 24, 2006. http://www.cbc.ca/news/background/workplace-safety/sick-workplace.html.

Centre for Equity in Health and Society (CEHS). http://www.beforequality.com/.

Chaska, N. 1978. "Status consistency and nurses= expectations and perception of role performance". *Nursing Research.* Vol. 27: 356-364.

_____ 1992. "The Staff nurse role". *Annual Review of Nursing Research.* Vol. 10: 185-201.

Chitty, K. K. 1997. *Professional: Concepts and Challenges.* Philadelphia: W. B. Saunders Co.

Coeling, H., & Cukr, P. 1997. "What's happening: Don't underestimate your collaboration skills." *Journal of the American Academy of Nurse Practitioners.* Vol. 9: 515-520.

College of Nurses of Ontario. 1995. "How Council Works". *Commuinqué.* Vol. 20 November.

College of Nurses of Ontario. 1995 (updated 1999). "Guidelines for Professional Behaviour". *Commuinqué.* Vol. 20 (1): 1-47.

College of Nurses of Ontario. 1995. "One is One Too Many. Prevention of Abuse of Clients; Expectations for Professional Behaviour". *Commuinqué.* Vol. 20(3) March.

College of Nurses of Ontario. 1996. "Role of CNO in Nursing Education". *Commuinqué.* Vol. 2(4): 34.

College of Nurses of Ontario. 1997. 'Protecting non-acute care". *Communiqué.* November. Vol. 22.

College of Nurses of Ontario. 1998 *Statistical database for Registered Nurses.* Fax on demand.

College of Nurses of Ontario. 1998. "Nursing with Styles: Forces of change move the profession forward". *Communiqué.* Vol. 23(3): 6-7.

College of Nurses of Ontario. 1998. "Issues? Discipline Committee: Protection to the Public, fairness to the nurse". *Commuinqué.* Vol. 30: 30.

College of Nurses of Ontario. 1998. "The Changing face of Nursing: Who are we?" *Commuinqué.* Vol. 23: 9-11.

College of Nurses of Ontario. 2004. *Registered Nurses Employed in Nursing in Ontario.* Membership Statistics Report, January 1, 2004.

College of Nurses of Ontario, 2004. *Nurse Abuse* Pub. No. 47004.

College of Nurses. *All About CNO.* http//www.cno.org/about.

College of Nurses. *A Spectrum of Service.* http://www.cno.org/upload/Spectrum.htlm.

Collins, E. et al., 1997-1998. *Research Toward Equity in the Professional Life of Immigrants: A Study of Nursing in the Metropolis* Toronto. (Research Report CERIS).

Collins, E., Hagey, R., Turrittin, J., Choudhry, U., Fudge, J. and Lee, R. 1999. *Study of Nursing in the Metropolis: Making racism See-able: the Grievances/complaints filed by women immigrant nurses of designated minority groups.* Toronto. (unpublished paper).

Cooks, Julie. 2000. *End The Silence* ZAC Films.

Corwin, R. G. 1961. "The professional employee: A study of conflict in nursing roles". *The American Journal of Sociology.* Vol. 66: 604-615.

Corwin, R. G. and Taves, M. J. 1962. "Some concomitants of bureaucratic and professional conceptions of the nurse role". *Nursing Research.* Vol. 22: 223-227.

Coudert, N., Fuchs, P. L., Roberts, C. S., Suhreinrich, J. A., and White, A. H. 1994. "Role Socialization of Graduating Student Nurses: Impact of a Nursing Practicum on Professional Role Conception". *Journal of Professional Nursing.* Vol. 10(6): 342-249.

Daily, R. 1988. "Head of nurses' group defends layoffs at Sick Kids". *The Toronto Star.* July 9. E3.

_____1998. "Nursing Care goes under the Microscope". *The Toronto Star.* August 10. A1.

_____1998. "Nurses seek to blacklist hospital". *The Toronto Star.* Aug. 25. B5.

Das Gupta, T. 1996. *Racism and Paid Work.* Toronto: Garamond Press.

_____ 1996. "Anti-Black Racism in Nursing in Ontario," *Studies in Political Economy.* Vol. 51(Fall): 97-116.

_____ 2002. *Racism in Nursing: Executive Summary* (Report). Toronto: Ontario Nurses Association.

_____ 2003."Racism in Nursing". http://www.ona.org/pdflib/dasgupta.pdf.

Denzin, N. K. 1989. *The Research Act: A Theoretical Introduction to Sociological Methods.* (3rd ed). Englewood Cliffs NJ: Prentice Hall.

Donner, G., Semogas, D., and Blythe, J. 1994. *Towards an Understanding of Nurses' Lives: Gender, Power, and Control.* Toronto. Quality of Nursing Worklife Research Unit. University of Toronto.

Dubin on Health Care. 1983. http://www.ontla.on.ca/hansard/committee_debates/36_parl/session1/estimates/e033.htm.

Duffin, C. 2002 "Racism in NHS is driving out ethnic minority nurses". *Nursing Standard.* Vol. 16(29): 4-5.

Duxbury, Linda and Chris Higgins. 2003. "Work-life Conflict in Canada in the New Millennium – A Status Report". Healthy Communities Division, Health Canada. http://www.phac-aspc.gc.ca/publicat/work-travail/pdf/rprt_2_e.pdf.

Essed, P. 1991. Understanding everyday racism: An interdisciplinary theory. Newbury Park, CA: Sage Publications.

Farr, M. 1991. "Discriminating Matters: There's more to racism than meets the eye". *The Registered Nurse.* February Vol. 3(1): 9-13.

Farrell, Gerald, A. 1997. "Aggression in clinical settings: nurses' views" *Journal of Advanced Nursing.* Vol. 25: 501-508.

Foucault. M. 1977. *Discipline and Power.* New York: Pantheon.

Freshwater, Dawn. 2000. "Crosscurrents: against cultural narration in nursing". *Journal of Advanced Nursing.* Vol. 32(2): 481.

Friedson, Eliot. 1990. "Professionalism, Caring, And Nursing." Paper prepared for The Park Ridge Center, Park Ridge, Illinois.

Gagnon, L. 1991. "Global Collegiality in Emergency nursing". *Journal of Emergency Nursing.* Vol. 17(1): 3.

Galabuzi, Grace-Edward. 2006. *Canada's Economic Apartheid: The Social Exclusion of Racialised Groups in the New Century.* Toronto: Canadian Scholars' Press Inc.

Glaser, B., and Strauss, A. 1973 [1967]. *The Discovery of Grounded Theory.* Chicago: Aldine.

Glazer, N., and Moyninhan, D. P. "Introduction". In Glazer, N. and Moyninhan, D. P. (Eds). *Ethnicity: Theory and Experience.* Cambridge: Harvard University Press.

Goffman, E. 1959. *The Presentation of Self in Everyday Life*. New York Doubleday Anchor.

_____ 1963 . *Behavior in Public Places*. Glencoe, Ill.: The Free Press.

Graydon, J. E., Kasta, W. and Khan, P. 1992. *The Personal and the Professional. Impact on the nurse of verbal and physical abuse* Nursing Innovation Fund. Ontario: Ministry of Health.

Greiner, L. E. 1972. "Evolution and revolution as organisations grow" *Harvard Business Review*. Vol. (4): 37-46.

Grow, S. J. 1991. *Who Cares? The Crisis in Canadian Nursing*. Toronto McClelland and Stewart Inc.

Hagey, R. 1999. What is racism? Culture Care Nursing Research Counci Publication. Toronto.

Hagey, R. and MacKay, R. 2000. "Qualitative research to identify racialis discourse: Towards equity in nursing curricula". *International Journal of Nursing Studies*. 37: 45-56.

Hagey, R., Lum, L., MacKay, R.,Turrittin, J., & Brody, E. 2001. *Exploring transformative justice in the employment of nurses: Toward recon- structing race relations and the dispute process*. Unpublished Report to the Law Commission of Canada.

Hagey et al. 2001. "Immigrant Nurses' Experience of Racism". *Journal o, Nursing Scholarship*. Vol. 33(4): 389-394.

Hagey, R., Turrittin, J., & Brody, E. 2002. "Antiracism advocacy in the climate of corporatization". In M. Jacobs (Ed.), *Is anyone listening? Women, Work, and Society*, pp. 315-335. Toronto: Women's Press.

Hagey, Rebecca, Jacobs, Merle, Turrittin, Jane, Purdy, Monica, Lee, Ruth, Cooper Brathwaite, Angela, Chandler, Marianne. 2005 *Implementing Accountability for Equity and Ending Racia. Backlash in Nursing:* Canadian Race Relation Foundation. http://www.crr.ca/Load.do?sectin=26&subSection=38&id=373&ty pe=2.

Hansen, H. 1995. "A model for Collegiality among Staff nurses in Acute care". *The Journal of Nursing Administration*. Vol. 25(12): 11-20.

Harper, T. 1998. "Nurses shortage a 'menace': Rock". *The Toronto Star*. June 16. A7.

Harrington, H. and Theis, C. 1968. "Institutional factors perceived by baccalaureate graduates as influencing their performance as staff nurses". *Nursing Research*. Vol. 25: 346-348.

Head, Wilson. 1985. *An exploratory study of the attitudes and perception of minority and majority health care workers*. Toronto: Ontario Ministry of Labour.

Health Services Restructuring Commission (HRCT). 1997. *A Vision of Ontario's Health Services System*. Jan. 1997.

Hill-Collins, P. 2000. *Black feminist thought: Knowledge, consciousness, and the politics of empowerment*. New York and London: Routledge.

Hospital Council on Metropolitan Toronto (HCMT). 1988. "Report of the HCMT Nursing Manpower Taskforce". Toronto.

Hughes, E. C., Hughes, H., and Deutscher, I. 1958. *Twenty Thousand Nurses Tell Their Story*. Montreal: J. B. Lippincott Company.

Hughes, E. C. 1958. *Men and their work*. New York: The Free Press.

Human Rights Commissions and Economic and Social Rights. Research Paper Policy and Education Branch. Toronto. Ontario Human Rights Commission. (website).

Hurst, J. B. and Keenan, M. (Photocopy)."Do you have any other ideas for improvement". *Nursing Success Today*. Vol. 23(1): 22-29.

Institute On Governance. 2001. *Ethnic Communities in Canada from a Governance Perspective: Unity in Diversity?* For The Transformations Program. http://www.iog.ca/publications/ethnic_communities.pdf.

Jacobs, M. 2000. "Staff Nurse Collegiality: The Structures, And Cultures That Produces Nursing Interactions". Unpublished doctoral dissertation, York University, Sociology.

_____ 2002. "Is anyone listening?: Women, Work, and Society." Toronto: Women's Press.

_____ 2006. "Nursing, A Pink Collar Ghetto? From Semi-Professional to Professional". In Jacobs, M. and Bosannac, Stephen, E. (Eds). *The Professionalization of Work*. Toronto: de Sitter Press.

Joint Policy and Planning Committee (JPPC) 1998. *Objectives*. http://www.jppc.org/mandate.htm.

Joint Policy and Planning Committee (JPPC). 1998. *An Overview*. http://www.jppc.org/jppc/stake.htm.

Johnson, D. 1959. "A philosophy of nursing". *Nursing Outlook* . Vol. 7: 198-200.

Jordan, S. 1983. "Collegiality in Nursing" *Orthopedic Nursing*. Vol. 2(3): 31-34.

217

Kilkus, S. P. 1990. "Self-Assertion and Nurses: A Different Voice". *Nursing Outlook*. Vol. 38(3): 145137-145143.

King, I. 1981. *A Theory for Nursing: Systems, Concepts, Process.* New York: Wiley

Kirby, S. and McKenna, K. 1989. *Methods from the Margins.* Toronto Garamond Press.

Kramer, M. 1968. "Role models, role conceptions, and role deprivation" *Nursing Research*. Vol. 17: 115-120.

_____ 1969. "Collegiate graduate nurses in medical center hospitals Mutual challenge of duel". *Nursing Research*. Vol. 18: 196-210.

_____ 1974. *Reality shock: Why nurses leave nursing.* St. Louis: C. V Mosby.

Letter. "If its nurses were unionized, Sick Kids would be blacklisted" by B Wahl (ONA President). *The Toronto Star*. July 17, A23.

Lowe, Graham, S. 2006. "Making a Measurable Difference: Evaluating Quality Worklife Interventions". Canadian Nurses Association www.cna-aiic.ca.

Lusk, S. L. 1992. "Violence experienced by nurses' aides in nursing homes An exploratory study". *AAOHN Journal*. Vol. 40(5): 237-241.

Mackay, L. 1989. *Nursing A Problem.* Stratford: Open University Press.

McGillis, Hall and Linda et al. 2003. "Indicators of Nurse Staffing and Quality Nursing Work Environments: A Critical Synthesis of the Literature". Faculty of Nursing, University of Toronto. Funded by the Ontario Ministry of Health & Long-Term Care.

McMahon, R. 1990. "Power and collegial relations among nurses on wards adopting primary nursing and hierarchical ward management structures". *Journal of Advanced Nursing*. Vol. 15: 232-239.

Millelstaedt, M. 1994. "Nurses get $320,000 in racism case". *The Globe and Mail*. May 13.

Ministry of Health. Ontario. 1999. *Good Nursing, Good Health: An Investment for the 21st Century.* wysiwyg://right.1/http//www gov.on.ca/h...ish/pub/ministyr/nurserep99/ profess.html.

Mitchell, S. 1971. "A women's profession: A man's research". Calgary University of Calgary.

Modibo, Najja Nwofia. 2004. "The Shattered Dreams of African Canadian Nurses". *Canadian Woman Studies/Les Cahiers De La Femme*. Vol. 23(2): 111-117.

218

Moloney, M. 1992. *Profession of Nursing* (2nd ed). Philadelphia: J. B. Lippincott Co.

Morgan, G. 1986. *Images of Organization*. Newbury Park: Sage Publications.

Muff, J. 1982. *Socialization, Sexism and Stereotyping*. St. Louis: The C.V. Mobsy Company.

Murrary, M. 1988a. *Nursing morale in Toronto*. Toronto: Hospital Council of Metropolitan Toronto (H.C.M.T. Report).

_____ 1988b. *Nursing resigning their hospital jobs in Toronto*. Toronto. Hospital Council of Metropolitan Toronto. (HCMT).

National Information Health Professionals. 1997. *Registered Nurses Employed in Nursing*. (Canada). http://www.cihi.ca/facts/canhr.htm.

Neugebauer, R. S. 1995. *Police - Community Relations: The Impact of Culture on the Control of Colour*. Unpublished doctoral dissertation, York University, Sociology.

Neuman, P. 1982. *The Neuman Systems Model* Norwalk, CT: Appleton-Lange.

Nolan, M. G. 1976. "Wanted: Colleagueship in Nursing". *Journal of Nursing Administration*. Vol. 6(3): 41-43.

Nursenet - A Global Forum for Nursing Issues. October, 31 1995. <NURSENET%UTORONTO.BITNET@UBVM.cc.buffalo.edu>.

Nursing Research. "Violence in Nursing: Study Confirms what most nurses know." *Registered Nurse*. Vol. 4(3): 20-21.

Nursing Times. 1990. "Are you a racist?" Questionnaire. April.

O'Brien-Pallas, Linda et al., 2004. "Evidence-based Standards for Measuring Nurse Staffing and Performance". Ontario Canadian Health Services Research Foundation. www.chrsf.ca.

O'Brien-Pallas, L., et al. 2004. "Evidence-Based Standards For Measuring Nurse Staffing &Performance". *FACT SHEET*, Nursing Health Services Research Unit. Funded by the Ontario Ministry of Health & Long-Term Care 2004-2009.

Ontario Hospital Association. 1994. Antiracism Report.

Ontario Hospital Association. Ontario Hospital Anti-Racism Taskforce Resource Package. 1996. Video, in conjunction with the package from the JPPC's "Anti-Racism Policy Guidelines Prepared by the Ontario Hospital Anti-racism Taskforce". Reference Document #4-2 (a) May 1996.

Ontario Hospital Association. 1998. *About Ontario Hospital Association* http//www.oha.com/oha/whawm.nsf/le2fl95...56bfca33493052563 000685329.

Ontario Hospital Association. "The Future of Health Care: A guide to the changes under way in Ontario" The Hospitals of Ontario (photo copy).

Ontario Hospital Association. 1977 "Redefining a Hospital". *Hospital Perspectives.* Vol. l4(3):3-7.

OHA Publications. "Guidelines for the Development of Hospital Policies on Managing Abuse". Ontario Hospital Association http://caohat03.oha.c0m/oha/ohapubl,nsf/...NoW.236?

OHA. Ontario Hospital Anti-Racism Taskforce Resource Package. 1996 Video, n conjunction with the package from the JPPC's "Anti Racism Policy Guidelines Prepared by the Ontario Hospital Anti-racism Taskforce". Reference Document #4-2 (a) May 1996.

Ontario Human Rights Commission. *Racial Harassment and Comment about a Person's Race.* Publication Ontario Human Right Commission.

Ontario Human Rights Commission. 2005. *Policy And Guidelines On Racism And Racial Discrimination.* http://www.ohrc.on.ca.

Ontario Human rights Commission Annual Report. 2005 .http://www.ohrc.on.ca/english/publications/2004-2005-annual report.shtml.

Ontario Nurses Association (ONA). 1988. *An Industry in Crisis: Ontario nurses speak out on the nursing shortage.* Position Paper. April.

Ontario Nurses Association (ONA). 1993. *Rethinking Health Care: Report on the State of Health Care in Ontario.* Toronto: ONA.

Ontario Nurses Association. 1994. Remarks by Ina Caissey. President Presentation to the City of North York's Community, Race and Ethnic Relations Committee. October 13.

Ontario Nursing Association. 1994. *From the President* (Remarks on Human Rights Commission). The ONA News. October. 3.

Ontario Nurses Association (ONA). 1996. *Dialogue on Health Reform: A Vision for Saving Medicare* Summer.

Ontario Nurses Association. 1996. *Government Policies Promote System Fragmentation.* http//www.ona.org/art-07.html.

Ontario Nurses Association. 1996. *Nurses want a meaningful voice in decision-making in the future system.* http//www.ona.org/art-04.html.

Ontario Nurses Association. *Queen's Park March.* Http//www.ona.org/march.html.

Ontario Nurses Association. *Realities Shared by Nurses, The Battle Ahead.* http//www.ona.org/art-09.html.

Ontario Nurses Association. "KISS: Keep it Simple Succinct: A practical approach to learning the initial steps of professional responsibility clause process". *Restructuring Bulletin.* http://www.ona/kiss.html.

Ontario Nurses Association (ONA). 1998. "Hospital Award Brings Gains For Ontario Nurses' Association Registered Nurses". *Media Release.* May 5, 1998.

Ontario Nurses Association. 1998. *Who We Are - What We Do.* http://222.ona.org/who.html.

Ontario Nurses Association. 1999 (updated 2005). Statement of Beliefs. "I'm Part of the Solution" (handbook for members).

Ontario Nurses Association Annual Report. 2003-2004. www.ona.org.

ONA *Visions.* 2003. "Racism in Nursing Study Undertaken". Vol. 30(2).

ONA Statement of Belief. 2005. http://www.ona.org/pdflib/pub_ statement_beliefs2005.pdf.

Ontario Nurses Association. 2006. Human Rights and Equity. *VISION.* Winter, Vol. 33(1):25.

Orem, D. M. 1985. *Nursing Concepts of Practice* (3rd ed). Englewood Cliffs: Prentice Hall.

Ornstein, M. 2000. *Ethno-Racial Inequality in the City of Toronto: An Analysis of the 1996 Census.* Toronto: City of Toronto.

Papp, L. 1994. "Seven nurses get award in landmark rights case". *The Toronto Star.* May 13.

Peplau, H. E. 1952. *Interpersonal Relations in Nursing.* New York: G. P. Putman's Sons.

Porter, J. 1965. *The Vertical Mosaic: An Analysis of Social Class and Power in Canada.* Toronto. University of Toronto Press.

Porter-O'Grady, T. 1991a. "Shared Governance for Nursing. Part1 Creating the New Organization". *AORN Journal.* Vol. 53(2): 458-466.

_____ 199b. "Shared Governance for Nursing. Part 2 Putting the Organization into Action". *AORN Journal.* Vol. 53(3): 694-703.

Poster, E. C. 1996. "A Multinational Study of Psychiatric Nursing Staff Beliefs and Concerns about Work Safety and Patient Assaults". *Archives of Psychiatric Nursing.* Vol. X(6): 365-373.

Priest, L. 1997. "Operating in the dark". *The Toronto Star*. September 20 A1.

_____ 1997. "Check up time". *The Toronto Star*. September 20. B1.

Prince, Althea and Susan Silva-Wayne. 2004. *Feminisms and Womanisms A Women's Studies Reader.* Toronto: Women's Press.

Puzan, Elayne. 2003. "The unbearable whiteness of being (in nursing)". *Nursing Inquiry*. Vol. 10(3): 193–200.

Randle, Jacqueline. 2003. "Bullying in the nursing profession". *Journal of Advanced Nursing*. Vol. 43(4): 395-401.

Registered Nurse. 1992." The End of the Nurse". April/May 13.

Reverby, S. 1987. "A caring dilemma: Womanhood and Nursing in Historical Perspective". *Nursing Research*. Vol. 36(1): 5-11.

RNAO. September 1994. *The Role of The Registered Nurse* http://www.rnal.org/po_st_13.htm.

RNAO *Action Alert: RNAO Advocacy Campaign* http://www.rnao.org aalert2.htm.

RNAO. 1994. "Racism in Nursing". *Remarks by Kathleen MacMillan President, RNAO*. September 13.

RNAO. 1996. *Statement on Cutbacks to the Hospital Sector* http//www.rnao.org/po_st_01.htm.

RNAO. 1997. *Nurses Join forces with Consumers to Tell the Story of Declining Standards of Health Care.* http//www.rnao.org/mr-11 6.html.

RNAO. 1998. "Political Election Platform". http://www..rnao.org elect.99.htm.

RNAO. 1998. *Shortage: Nursing Week the state of Nursing in Ontario* http//www.rnao.org/nr_ar_43.htm.

RNAO. 2002. *Tracking the Nursing Task Force (1999): RNs Rate Their Nursing Work Life.* www.rnao.org.

RNAO *Report to the Board for the period May 15, 2004 – August 31, 2004.*

RNAO Revised: September 2004. Healthy Work Environments Best Practice Guidelines Organizational Chart. Project Team funded Health Canada.

RNAO. 2005. *Woman abuse: screening, identification and initial response* Toronto. ON.

Registered Nurses Association of Ontario. Joint Statement. *Replacement of Registered Nurses by Less Prepared Providers.* http//www. rnao.org/po-st-04.html.

Ritzer, George. 1990. *Frontiers of Social Theory: The New Syntheses.* New York: Columbia University Press.

Roberts, S. 1991 "Nurse Abuse: A Taboo Topic". *The Canadian Nurse.* Vol. 87(3): 23-25.

Ross, A. D. 1961. *Becoming a Nurse.* Toronto: The Macmillian Co. of Canada.

Roth, J. 1982. *Research in the Sociology of health Care: Changing structure of health service occupations.* Greenwich Connecticut: JAI Press Inc.

Roth, R. 1995. "Collegiality in nursing and all-pro football games". *AORN Journal.* Vol. 41(2): 326-328.

Rounds, K. 1993. "Report from the Wards: Nurses Speak Out". *Ms Magazine.* January/February 34-36.

Roy, C. 1983. *Introduction to Nursing: An Adaptation Model* (2nd ed). Englewood Cliffs: Prentice Hall.

Ryan, J. and E. C. Poster. 1991. "When a Patient hits you". *The Canadian Nurse.* Vol. 87(8): 23-29.

Samuel, Edith. 2005. *Integrative Antiracism: South Asians in Canadian Academe.* Toronto: University of Toronto Press.

Singleton, E. K., and F. C. Nail. 1984. "Role clarification: A prerequisite to autonomy". *The Journal of Nursing Administration.* Vol. 14(10):17-22.

Spicer, J., Gygax Ripple, H. B., Louie, E., Baj, P., Keating. S. 1994. "Supporting Ethnic and Cultural Diversity in Nursing Staff". In *Nursing Management.* Vol. 25(1): 38-40.

Squires, T. 1995. "Men in Nursing". *Registered Nurse.* July 26-28.

Statistics Canada. *Visible minority population, 1996 Census.* http://www.statcan.ca:80/english/Pgdb/People/Population/demo40f .htm.

Statistics Canada. *Immigrant population, by place of birth, 1996 Census.* http;//www.statcan.ca:80/english/Pgdb/People/Population/demo35f .htm.

Street, A. F. 1992. *Inside Nursing.* New York: State University of New York Press.

Styles, M. 1982. *On Nursing.* St. Louis: The Mobsy Co.

Suryamani, E. 1989. *The Organization and the Semi-professional.* New Delhi: Jainsons Publications.

Taves, M. V., Corwin, R. G. and Haas, J. E. 1963. *Role Conception and vocational success and satisfaction: A Study of Student and Professional Nurses.* Columbus: The Ohio State University.

223

Taylor, Bev. 2001. "Identifying and transforming dysfunctional nurse-nurse relationships through reflective practice and action research" *International Journal of Nursing Practice*. Vol. 7: 406-413.

The Toronto Star. (Chicago Trubune. By Mary Sue Mohnke) 1991. "It's okay to put yourself first, nurse says". December 12, D18.

The Toronto Star. 1998. Editorial: "Open all hospitals to public scrutiny" June, 30. E2.

Travelbee, J. 1977. [1966] *Interpersonal Aspects of Nursing*. 2nd edition F.A. Davis Company.

Turner, R. 1977. In. W. Metzger (ed) *Reader of the Sociology of the Academic Profession*. New York: ARNO Press.

United Nations Committee on Economic, Social and Cultural Rights, *Fact Sheet No. 16 (Rev. 1)(1991)*, online: United Nations Office of the High Commissioner for Human Rights Homepage http://www.unhchr.ch/html/menu6/2/fs16.htm.

Vance, C.M. 1977. *A group profile of contemporary influentials in American nursing*. Doctoral dissertation, Columbia University Teachers College, New York, New York.

Visano, L.A. 1987. *This Idle Trade*. Concord, ON: Vistasna.

_____ 2006. *What Do They Know? Youth, Crime and Culture*. Toronto: de Sitter Publications.

Wagner, E. J. 1992. *Sexual Harassment in the Workplace*. New York AMACON, American Management Association.

Weber, M. 1946. "Class, Status and Party". In Gerth, H. and Mills, C. W (Eds). *From Max Weber: Essays is Sociology* New York: Oxford Press.

Williams, C. L. 1995. "Hidden advantages for men in nursing". *Nursing Administration Quarterly*. Vol. 19(2): 63-70.

Wolf, Z. 1988a. *Nurses' work: The sacred and the profane*. Philadelphia University of Pennsylvania.

_____ 1988b. "Nursing Rituals". *The Canadian Journal of Nursing Research*. Vol. 20(3): 59-69.

Wuest, J. 1994. "Professionalism and the Evolution of Nursing as a discipline: A Feminist Perspective". *Journal of Professional Nursing* Vol. 10(6): 357-367.

Index

225

185, 206
Professionalization, 85, 91, 92, 95, 97
Promotions, 100, 114
Puzan, Elayne, 76, 100, 222
Quinn, C., 211
Race, 1, 9, 12, 17, 20, 93, 104, 142, 144, 196, 197, 204, 206, 207, 209
Racialised, 1, 2, 5, 8, 9, 14, 15, 16, 18, 19, 21, 22, 31, 36, 37, 38, 39, 53, 54, 55, 93, 100, 103, 110, 114, 115, 116, 118, 120, 134, 141, 142, 143, 144, 160, 164, 174, 175, 176, 181
Racism, 1, 2, 3, 4, 5, 6, 7, 10, 11, 12, 13, 14, 15, 16, 17, 18, 19, 20, 21, 30, 31, 36, 46, 49, 50, 53, 54, 55, 93, 94, 96, 100, 110, 115, 116, 118, 120, 126, 134, 141, 142, 143, 144, 148, 149, 150, 160, 164, 170, 173, 174, 175, 176, 181, 183, 186, 188, 189, 190, 192, 193, 204, 205, 206, 209
Randle, Jacqueline, 222
Registered Nurse (RN), 38, 39, 43, 57, 58, 62, 63, 72, 74, 75, 77, 79, 80, 82, 83, 84, 86, 88, 91, 92, 132, 136, 215, 219, 222, 223
Registered Nurses Association of Ontario (RNAO), 6, 7, 8, 15, 27, 41, 57, 58, 59, 60, 61, 62, 67, 74, 75, 76, 78, 79, 80, 82, 83, 85, 86, 87, 88, 89, 92, 96, 97, 99, 103, 108, 114, 116, 123, 125, 137, 142, 143, 155, 176, 183, 194, 222.
Registered Practical Nurses (RPN) 38, 39, 70, 76
Relationships, 93, 96, 114, 115, 127, 128
Respect, 152, 153, 154, 155, 156, 157, 177, 178
Reverby, S., 96, 222

RHPA, 62, 64, 85
Risk-taking, 163, 164, 165, 166, 169, 178
Ritzer, George, 61, 223
Roberts, S., 223
Ross, A.D., 34, 96, 137, 223
Roth, J., 25, 223
Roth, R., 223
Rounds, K., 22, 23, 223
Roy, C., 98, 99, 223
Ryan, J., 223
Samuel, Edith, 14, 223
SARS, 66
Sexism, 3, 183, 192, 205
Sexual harassment, 1
Sexual orientation, 209
Sinclair, Duncan, 77, 78
Social justice, 1, 6, 9, 10, 14, 20, 21, 24, 40, 93, 183, 184, 186, 190, 194, 202, 205, 208, 210
Squires, T., 36, 223
Staff nurse 14, 16, 20, 21, 22, 24, 27, 28, 29, 30, 31, 32, 33, 35, 36, 37, 38, 39, 42, 43, 44, 45, 46, 47, 48, 50, 54, 58, 59, 61, 62, 63, 65, 66, 67, 69, 70, 71, 73, 74, 76, 77, 78, 79, 80, 81, 83, 85, 86, 88, 89, 90, 91, 92, 93, 94, 95, 97, 98, 99, 101, 102, 103, 104, 105, 106, 107, 108, 109, 111, 112, 113, 115,116, 117, 118, 119, 120, 121, 122, 123, 124, 125, 126, 127, 128, 129, 130, 131, 132, 133, 134, 135, 136, 137, 138, 139, 140, 141, 143, 145, 146, 148, 149, 150, 151, 153, 154, 155, 156, 157, 158, 160, 161, 162, 163, 164, 165, 166, 167, 168, 169, 170, 171, 172, 173, 176, 177, 178, 179, 180, 181, 183, 184, 185, 186, 187, 188, 190, 191, 192, 193,

230

Printed in the United States
65588LVS00005B/1-75